A Guide to
Natural Health Care

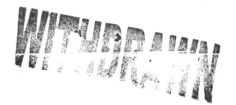

Also by the same author

A Guide to Precision Reflexology

*He who... can no longer feel amazement, is as good as dead,
a snuffed-out candle.*

Albert Einstein

A Guide to
Natural Health Care

Jan Williamson

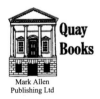

Quay
Books

Mark Allen
Publishing Ltd

Quay Books Division, Mark Allen Publishing Ltd, Jesses Farm, Snow Hill, Dinton, Salisbury, Wiltshire, SP3 5HN

British Library Cataloguing-in-Publication Data
A catalogue record is available for this book

© Mark Allen Publishing Ltd 2001
ISBN 1 85642 187 2

Printed in the UK by Bath Press, Bath

Contents

Acknowledgements   vii

Foreword   ix

Introduction   xi

1   What is natural health care?   1

2   Reflexology   5

3   Yoga   21

4   Relaxation and rest   36

5   Nutrition   44

6   Massage   56

7   Pregnancy and post-natal care   73

Review – how to use this book   89

Summary   95

Recommended reading list and useful addresses   97

Index   99

Acknowledgements

Thank you to Susan, Lesley, Ali, Faith, Sue, Alison, Kerry and Lula for your help with the photographs and also to PK Photography.

Dedication

To friendship...

Foreword

Jan Williamson's considerable experience as a practitioner, teacher and researcher of complementary health illumines the pages of this friendly book. In fact, she has successfully managed to make even the most potentially mystifying aspects of complementary health 'user-friendly'.

Jan achieves this by stressing a consistent theme, a focus which is often overlooked in the search to experience natural health methods and techniques – that each one of us is our own health expert. She offers an integrated view which puts the emphasis on individuality as the 'natural'. This approach encourages the reader to search for personal meaning in what complementary health has to offer, and creates a more enlightened attitude towards the need to take responsibility for our own health.

Jan delivers her message wisely in how she explains in detail the complementary spirit of natural health care. She illustrates the benefits of following natural methods while reminding us that it is not the sole aim of complementary health to live a life without pain. I am impressed with her assertion that health is 'not always about being well'. She draws from her clinical experience in pointing out that our state of health often tends to reflect life situations, and guides the reader towards a deeper appreciation of well being.

Jan's deep commitment clearly comes from an in-depth study of the wider implications of health care, which balances the social and spiritual aspects of life. For this, she presents the relevance of disciplines such as yoga to emphasise the necessity for rest and reflectiveness, and the role of the massage therapies, including her own speciality, Reflexology, in building confidence and trust. The value of other therapies is confirmed in extensive referencing throughout the book, which is not always available in a work of this kind.

I am happy to congratulate Jan on the publication of *A Guide to Natural Health Care*. This book extends her reliable guidance to a wider public and I am sure it will be warmly received.

Stewart Mitchell
Exeter, September 2000

Introduction

Individuality of care

There are genuine possibilities for complementary health care to have a place in everyone's life if they would like it to be there; this book offers suggestions for ways to achieve this. It will depend on individual personality, need and lifestyle which approach is the most attractive to you. The choice you make needs to feel comfortable and appropriate. Each reader will relate to some aspects more than others. The individuality of this choice is important and is, in fact, central to the treatment itself and will have a direct bearing on the benefits which can be achieved.

Enjoy looking after yourself!

The initial involvement and participation offers the opportunity to be creative and imaginative; this is often a pleasant surprise allowing, as it does, health care to be an enjoyable process.

User-friendly care

The first step is often the most difficult but, if this is the case, it may be helpful to consider firstly, that complementary care is supportive and friendly. It is not remote but rather it is available for everyone to some degree or other. Secondly, it can also offer ways to look after yourself as much, or as little, as you choose. A variety of approaches can be used and the ones described in this book are complementary to each other and can safely be used together. This book gives:

* An overview of a range of therapies. What to expect from them and when to use them.

* Relevant self-help advice with practical applications.

* What complementary health care can mean to each person. How it can be applied to everyday situations and stages in life. Advice on ways to look after self.

* A multi-faceted approach. Each reader will be attracted more to one approach than another. Advice on how to use several approaches in conjunction with each other.

Aims of the book

* To increase confidence and trust with the use and application of complementary health care techniques.

* To offer realistic guidelines so that each person can 'fit' the suggestions into their world, as they wish.

* To de-mystify the world of complementary care – traditionally natural therapies were based in the home environment and not in 'ivory towers'.

* To increase awareness and understanding of how the body functions and to relate this to our emotional and physical health. To show how this knowledge need not seem daunting but rather it is an instinctive process, engendering a sense of great self-respect and wonderment.

* To demonstrate how health care can be an enjoyable experience.

* To show how becoming more involved with our own health care can be a process of positive change and personal growth.

Appropriate health care

There are aspects of this approach to health care that can suit the individual in a friendly and adaptable way. For example, it is often helpful to recommend rest: for one person this may be experienced by practising an advanced yoga posture such as the shoulderstand and, for another person, the same benefits can be achieved by sitting in their favourite armchair and putting their feet up on a stool. Or one person, at different times in their life, may choose to adopt one of these techniques in preference to the other. It is not a case of one approach being better than the other, or of one being second best, or even that one is a modification to be practised until the other can be achieved but, rather, that the method 'matches' the person at that time – on all levels of their being.

It may be that the therapies are used purely and simply as care management based in the home with, perhaps, a practitioner being involved from time to time. Or it may be that the focus is on the professional consultations, with some home care to extend the benefits of the treatment sessions. Choose whatever feels right at the time for you – you know best.

1

What is natural health care?

This book is an attempt to place complementary therapy within the context of each reader's everyday existence, and to explain the meaning of this approach to health care in **reality**.

The initial enquiry

The concept of natural or complementary health is now a familiar one, receiving as it does so much media attention. It may sound very attractive but this is meaningless unless it has a relevance to daily life.

The situation is further complicated by the seemingly confusing array of therapies on offer. Questions which naturally arise from this include ones such as:

What do all these therapies mean?	What will happen in the consultation?
How can each one help me?	How much will it cost?
Which one should I choose?	How will I feel afterwards?

Which is the right one for me?

Here are some general ideas to consider about natural health care:

* First of all you don't need to be ill to receive complementary care – there is real value to be had from using the treatment to maintain good health. As you develop a greater understanding of your own health issues you can use this approach in a preventative way.

* This approach to health care doesn't need to be expensive or exclusive although, at first sight, it may seem like this. With increased understanding and awareness comes confidence to manage some aspects of health yourself. This self-help approach makes the economic prospects of complementary care more attractive. It is not an exclusive regime, in fact, the traditions of natural therapy are derived from home care with the techniques being handed down through the generations. In this way it is possible for each individual to take from complementary care elements that are acceptable to them.

* There is no question of appraisal or judgement with the way each person chooses to care for themselves. You can take what you need and **you know best**. It can be used as a total health system in itself or alongside allopathic care – as long as all care professionals involved are informed.

* Each person is their own health care expert. You know yourself better than anyone else.

* Being involved with complementary care isn't about being well all the time. It is about attempting to **understand** health and illness, striving to see the message behind the illness and responding to it in a positive manner. This involves seeing it as a time to learn and grow within a supportive environment. Adopting this approach means that it is never a wasted time nor a time of denial but an opportunity to respond to what your body needs.

The first, and most important question for most people is, 'which therapy to choose?' There is no one single definitive answer because complementary care deals with **real people**, each one with their own ability, culture, lifestyle and, as a result, their own preferences. But, of course, we all need some guidance and advice about how to make this choice. With this in mind, here are some points to consider:

* Which therapy do I feel drawn to? We all have natural personal preferences. With knowledge that you already have, which one appeals to you?

* Resource people around you. Ask them: Do they receive any natural therapies? What can they tell you about the practitioner? What happens in the treatment? Has it helped? Personal recommendation is always the most valuable information.

* While all complementary therapies focus on the whole person, rather than on the specific condition, it is often a particular symptom that prompts someone to explore a new approach to health care and this often helps with the decision-making. For instance, it may be more appropriate to have a 'hands-on' therapy rather than one which is totally consultative. So the choice may depend on your overall state of health at the time – this may be emotional or physical health.

* Obviously you need to check out the practitioner's experience and skill. It is absolutely appropriate to ask what qualifications they have and to which professional body they belong.

The importance of the choice of practitioner

A vital element in receiving complementary health care is the relationship that can be established between the practitioner and the recipient of the treatment. Ideally, over a period of time, there develops an atmosphere of mutual trust and respect. This is dependent on the personalities involved and usually our intuition can be relied on to assess this at the initial consultation. This relationship is often the support needed as people begin to explore the world of complementary care and to develop their own health care skills. It gives time to be listened and attended to, and can be used as a reference point when acquiring skills to manage a new health care regime.

The meaning of being unwell

Complementary health care supports **reality**, with real people in life situations. It recognises that as individuals we all have varying degrees of commitment. The richness of life is that human beings are sociable creatures and this fact brings with it many positive features, but also, some negative ones. Complications in our lives are often centred around other people.

Natural health care supports the process of illness and health existing side-by-side. It acknowledges that illness is part of health and not separate from it, not something to be seen as alien. We have just one health which is constantly adapting and responding to our world. We cannot separate our state of health from the world that we choose to inhabit; it affects and is affected by whatever constitutes that world. Factors which relate to our health include relationships, career, nutrition, climate, culture, background, heredity, disposition, exercise, the environment, everything in fact which makes up our lifestyle. Often there is a challenge to be faced as we recognise that changes need to be made. Natural health care does not deny nature and it does not deny the symptom. We have to accept that often nature is unkind, a fact that we are all aware of when we consider the world of animals. This acceptance implies a sense of reality, not of suppression. There is a misconception that therapies are the softer option being purely and simply about relaxation – this may sometimes be the case and there is real value to that – but often there is much more in terms of exploring the situation and achieving a level of understanding.

The professional consultations can provide a situation for the individual recipient to get to know themselves better, for them to express their concerns and to be listened to. Each person can feel involved in, and aware of, their own health to whichever level feels right for them. This increased understanding can be achieved by accepting that, if there is a problem, it is a part of them, not something alien and, as such, it is possible to attach meaning to the process. This acceptance does not mean being defeated but instead it offers a positive way forward. One important aspect in complementary care is that the symptom is not necessarily the focus of the treatment, but rather the person who has that symptom is the centre of attention. Initially this may be a new and possibly difficult concept, but it offers a positive outlook for the future. An example of this would be to consider two people who are both anxious and suffering from stress, and who are unwell as a result. One has developed eczema and the other has digestive problems. They are each unwell in their own way, each symptom obviously needs to be addressed but the long-term approach would be to look at ways that they can each reduce the stress in their lives. This will most probably involve a different management plan for each of them depending on their lifestyle and personal preferences. The initial idea that a symptom which is perhaps unpleasant, painful or debilitating can be accepted as a friend may seem absurd and, understandably, often needs time and lots of support in order to become tolerable. The forum of the consultation with your practitioner can provide this time and support. Perhaps we should be grateful to the symptom because it draws our attention to ourselves and it is the body's way of saying that it is not well and needs some care. An example of this process of acceptance is the all too familiar headache scenario, a painkiller provides a welcome relief and a 'quick-fix' but it doesn't prevent the headache from reoccurring when a similar situation arises. It suppresses the actual symptom but actually prolongs the condition and, all too often, it worsens as the headache increases in intensity each time. Instead, the more holistic approach would be to ask what causes the headache and then to address these issues. This challenge will take longer than the 'quick-fix' but will ultimately be more positive. The causes can be many and varied; these could include dietary conditions, hormonal imbalances, postural problems, stressful situations or environmental issues. These situations can then be addressed either by means of the therapy, by making realistic lifestyle changes and/or by using self-help techniques. Or, on a more psychological level, it may be relevant to see the headache as a way of the body, and the mind, taking some 'time-out'. If this seems relevant then perhaps it is appropriate to consider if the rest can be provided in more pleasant ways or even to make changes so that the need for the rest is reduced at source. This involvement recognises that each person is their own health expert – they know their own strengths and weaknesses, they know the things that make them anxious, enthusiastic, happy or sad. This approach provides support as each individual's confidence grows and they can learn to trust their own judgement more and more.

The learning process can also mean that you may look at health issues from a wider perspective, from a different point of view. Two examples of illness to illustrate this are:

Infections: The most effective care for any infection is to be able to rest and we are all familiar with the scenario of not taking long enough to recover from an illness and then it returns. However, it is usually much worse the second time. We can translate this into seeing an infection as the body's way of saying that it needs to rest.

High blood pressure: It is acceptable to see that this may be caused by external factors, a response to stressful situations, but it is also worth considering that it may be as a result of internal factors such as the nature and quantity of food and drink that the body has to process. This can be such that it overworks all the body functions, creating inappropriate pressure.

This more lateral approach can influence the manner of future health care in a sensible, logical way.

Unique nature of natural therapy

Sickness is not an accident, it is not an isolated event but rather it is the way in which the body communicates with itself and with the world around it. In the same way that complementary health care accepts that we all have our own unique set of circumstances which affect, and which are affected by, our health, it also states that we each have our own way of responding to health issues. Just as the influences differ so also must the involvement in, and nature of, future health care. Health care programmes differ from one person to another and from one set of circumstances to another, being a response to that individual at that particular time. Certain lifestyle changes may be necessary in order to progress but these must be changes that the person is ready to make. Any care plan needs to be within realistic limits. There may be aspects of it that present a challenge but these will undoubtedly bring the most rewards.

To continue...

The following chapters show, in practical ways, how natural therapy can be used for health care, both professionally and in the home environment.

2
Reflexology

Rationale for reflexology

While the practice of reflexology is a relatively recent development in the field of complementary therapy in the Western world, it is an ancient holistic healing technique derived from oriental philosophy. This philosophy believes that when someone is not well, their energy system – the part of them that makes them unique – is out of balance. The aim of reflexology, along with other holistic therapies, is to connect to a person's energy, to adjust it and harmonise it with the world in which that person lives. In human beings this energy is physical, emotional and spiritual, it is a dynamic system and it is constantly changing.

Reflexology is a form of foot (and sometimes hand) massage and the belief is that there is a reflex area on the feet for every part of the body. Practitioners believe that by applying pressure to the feet, it is possible to connect to the relevant areas of the body. The physical connections are via the nervous and circulatory systems and the healing process is to nourish and heal by stimulating the circulation to the appropriate body part. The treatment has a beneficial effect on the nervous system thus promoting deep relaxation and providing an optimum situation for the restoration of health.

Reflexology can have a positive effect in its ability to relieve stress and tension, be it physical or emotional. It does not offer a diagnosis but, rather, it can be seen as a form of examination which can contribute to an understanding of a condition.

History

The feet have held a special place in history, mythology and cultures throughout the world. In mythology the famous reference is that of Achilles' heel, meaning a vulnerable area. The removal of shoes at the threshold of holy places for the Buddhists, the Hindus and the Muslims is compulsory. Among reflexologists it is a widely held theory that reflexology originated in China some 5000 years ago, and there is Egyptian documentation dating from around 2500–2300 BC. In the tomb of Ankhmahor, a highly respected physician, there are wall paintings showing what appears to be the practice of reflexology (see *Figure 2.1*). The origins of reflexology are in ancient history when pressure therapies were recognised and accepted as preventative and therapeutic.

There has been an acceleration of interest in the West since the turn of the twentieth century when an American doctor, Dr William Fitzgerald, 'discovered' reflexology while travelling through Europe. He went on to use the therapy in the management of pain, applying pressure to specific points on the feet and hands while conducting minor operations without the need for anaesthetic. This work was further developed by colleagues in America and then, finally, brought over to Britain in 1966 by a practitioner called Doreen Bayly. Since then it has become increasingly popular and it is now recognised as a valid form of complementary therapy.

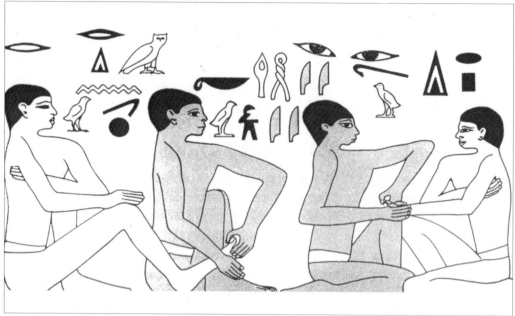

Figure 2.1: Wall paintings from the tomb of Ankhmahor

The treatment

Reflexologists believe that the feet represent the energy of the body. For example, it is believed that the big toe corresponds to the head (see *Figure 2.2*). The reflex for the spine is located on the inside edge of each foot. The reflex areas for the organs and structures of the right side of the body are on the right foot and those of the left side are on the left foot (see *Figure 2.3*). The reflex areas are on both the sole and the top of the foot. The same principles apply to the hands (see *Figure 2.4*) .

In the professional setting, practitioners are trained to respond to each treatment with a variety of specific thumb and finger techniques, and to develop sensitivity, so that each consultation is conducted in a thoroughly caring and responsible way. In addition to their reflexology training, they have an extensive knowledge of the anatomy and physiology of the body. As well as the skill and expertise of the practitioner, within the consultation, there is the additional benefit of having the exclusive time and attention of the practitioner.

As pressure is applied to different reflex areas on the feet, or hands, different sensations will be felt. Reactions differ from one person to another and from one treatment to another; each treatment being a response to that person, at that time. One person may feel energised and another may feel deeply relaxed. The treatment does not focus on a symptom but rather on the person who has the symptom. Reflexology is one way, among many, of having time for yourself, time to reflect, to relax, to try to understand any health problems and to try to find some meaning behind them. Rather than simply controlling symptoms, the ethos is to work with the body and to progress accordingly.

Recipients commonly express feelings of improved well-being. The majority of patients find that the treatment reduces stress-related disorders, helping them to cope better with the pressures of everyday life.

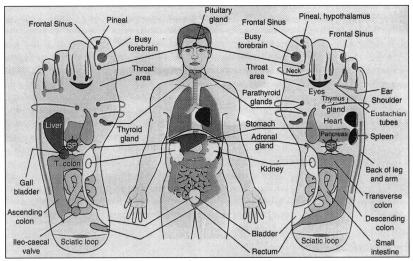

Figure 2.2: Reflex areas of the feet, with the body parts to which they correspond

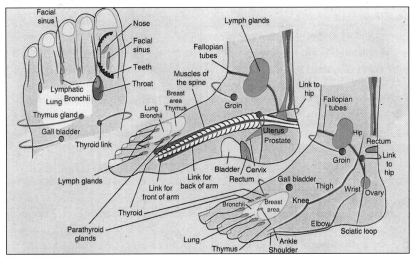

Figure 2.3: Reflex areas of the feet, showing their symmetry

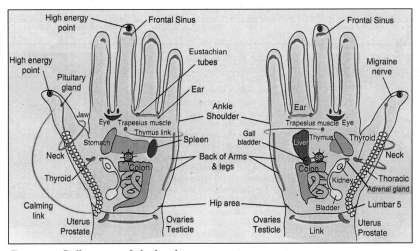

Figure 2.4: Reflex areas of the hands

Precision reflexology

This is one form of the therapy which particularly resonates with the Eastern philosophical approach. It uses a technique which connects to the energy of a person and aims to support the patient as they themselves strive to restore balance to the system. This technique is described in detail in *A Guide to Precision Reflexology* (1999).

Home care with reflexology

In addition to professional treatments, reflexology with its ease of availability, can readily be used in the home environment, either as self-help or to treat family and friends. No special equipment is needed , you just need someone's feet and your hands. As long as both people are comfortable, it is not essential to use special treatment couches or chairs. It can be adapted to a variety of settings, a quiet room indoors, under the shade of a tree on a sunny day or even on a train journey after a busy day!

Practitioners often advise self-help techniques to use in-between sessions in order to reinforce the benefits of the professional treatment. Also, there are occasions when home care can be valuable as a 'first aid' skill or to treat minor problems. Quite apart from the physical benefits, the knowledge that in certain situations, you have the skill and confidence to look after yourself, can be enormously valuable.

Using either the hands or the feet there is much that can be achieved in terms of management of your own health care. Reflexology is a totally non-invasive therapy. It is possible to adjust and re-adjust the responses on many reflexology points using your own body in a self-contained manner. Much of the appeal of this therapy is its simplicity and accessibility. By feeling the sensitivity of these responses and the effect that they can have on your own health, you become aware of the connections throughout your physical and emotional self. Our hands and feet reflect what is happening elsewhere in the body. In this way you learn both to trust your own instincts and to be amazed by the accuracy of the innate intelligence of your own body. This approach leads to increased confidence and, subsequently, increased trust. In a very practical 'hands-on' way you can learn to listen to yourself and respond accordingly.

All of the following procedures can be used in isolation as quick remedies when needed. For additional relaxation benefit they can also be combined within a foot massage sequence (see *Chapter 6, pp. 58–62*).

Headache treatment

Foot treatment – Apply gentle circular pressure with the thumb to the area on the big toe pad indicated in *Figure 2.5*. In cases of severe pain, this will be very sensitive and so modify the amount of pressure used. Work the area for one minute, use gentle foot massage techniques to ease the headache by promoting relaxation and then repeat.

It is advisable to treat both feet, if one feels more sensitive than the other, then pay more attention to the sensitive one.

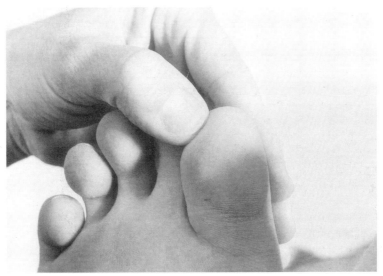

Figure 2.5

Hand treatment – Apply gentle circular thumb pressure to the relevant area on the thumb, see *Figure 2.6*. As for the foot, intersperse this with massage (*p.58*). Repeat for the other hand.

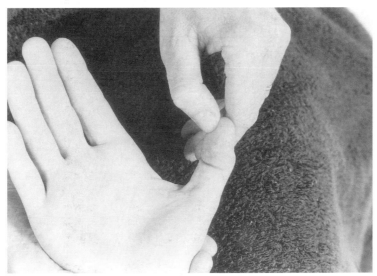

Figure 2.6

Neck pain and tension

Foot treatment – Using firm circular pressure work all around the base of the big toe. See *Figure 2.7*. In the same way that you can feel tension when you massage someone's neck, it is possible to feel it here too and this stroke can be used to ease out this strain.

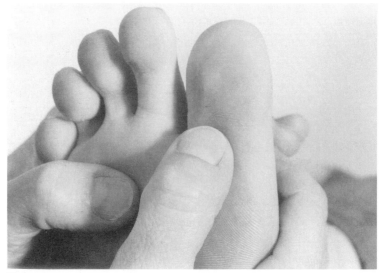

Figure 2.7

Hand treatment – Using firm circular pressure work all around the base of the thumb. See *Figure 2.8*.

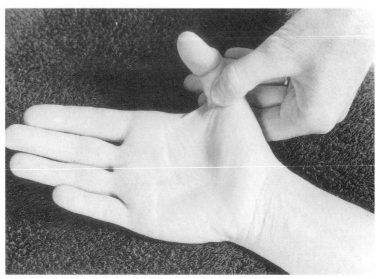

Figure 2.8

Sore throats

Foot treatment – The reflex area for the throat is located on the top of the foot, in the space between the big toe and the second toe. Use a firm smoothing stroke to work the area from the base of the toes towards the ankle, locating sensitive areas. *See Figure 2.9*. Use a gentle circular pressure on any sensitive spots.

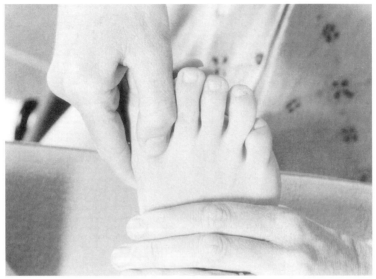

Figure 2.9

Hand treatment – This is in a corresponding area on the hand, in the web between the thumb and the forefinger. Use a firm smoothing stroke from the base of the thumb towards the wrist. See *Figure 2.10*.

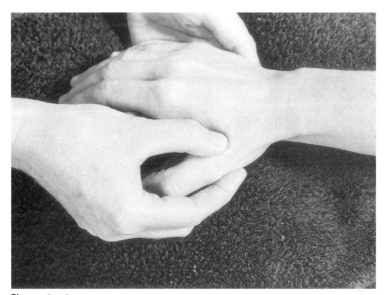

Figure 2.10

Sinusitis

Foot treatment – These reflexes are located around the edge of each toe and it is possible to experience great relief from the pain and congestion of this condition by using reflexology. People report maximum benefit if treatment can be administered at the first indication of the problem. Alternating between the middle finger and thumb for convenience, use a circular pressure around each toe. See *Figure 2.11*. It is possible to feel the congestion around these areas, which usually presents itself as gritty areas to touch. Use a degree of caution for acute conditions because this will be quite painful, if this is the case, then intersperse the treatment with lots of foot massage. Each time you return to the area, you will find that you can apply more pressure to be more effective. The amount of pressure used needs to be appropriate to the related body part. The sinuses are delicate cavities so it needs to be a definite pressure so as not to be ticklish but it should not be too invasive.

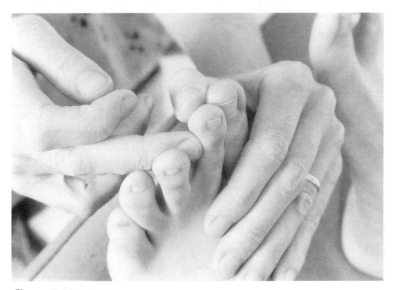

Figure 2.11

Hand treatment – These reflexes are located around the edge of each finger. See *Figure 2.12*. As with the toes, use a circular pressure around the outline of each finger. Greater attention can be given to areas of greater sensitivity. People report great relief from using this self-help technique, often being able to reduce prescribed medication under the guidance of their physician. The easy accessibility of the hands means that the treatment can take place on a 'little and often' basis for maximum benefit. It can be carried out almost anywhere, for instance at the office desk, while waiting for a train or when watching television.

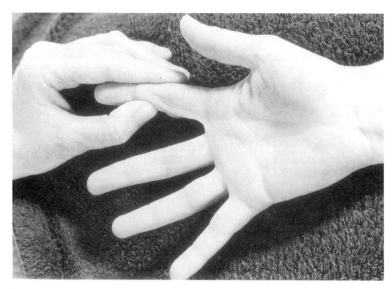

Figure 2.12

Pain relief

Foot treatment – The nervous system is the way in which we register and respond to pain and the solar plexus is a network of nervous activity in the centre of the body. The reflex for this area is situated in the centre of the sole of the foot. See *Figure 2.13*. To ease pain anywhere in the system, apply gentle circular pressure to this point. This needs to feel comfortable and supportive, so be sensitive to the level of pain present and match the pressure accordingly.

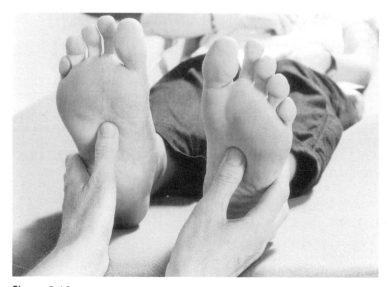

Figure 2.13

Hand treatment – Again corresponding to the feet, the solar plexus reflex is in the centre of the palm of the hand. See *Figure 2.14*. Apply pressure to this area with the thumb of the other hand to assist with pain relief. This same method can be used to **reduce nervous tension in stressful situations**. This is particularly relevant with the hands because of the free accessibility. It is possible to become aware of the integration of the body as you can feel yourself becoming calmer and more still. This is further enhanced with the addition of the deep breathing technique as described in *Chapter 3 (p. 32)*. The advantage being that this 'tool' is totally portable and can be applied wherever you are.

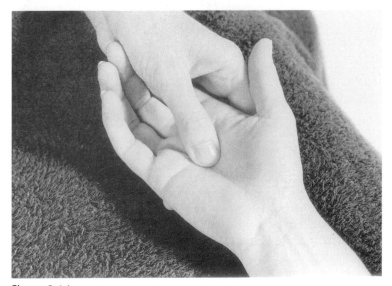

Figure 2.14

Constipation

Foot treatment – To address this problem in the long-term, a multi-faceted approach is required, involving the issues of relaxation, diet and exercise. However, it is possible to obtain short-term relief with the application of reflexology. The reflex area for the colon, the large intestine, is spread over both feet and a deep circular pressure needs to be applied along it's full length. See *Figure 2.15*. Tension in this area can be felt via the reflex.

Hand treatment – The reflex is spread over both hands. See *Figure 2.16*. Once again, a deep pressure needs to be applied along it's length.

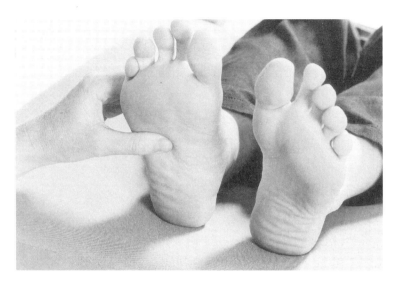

Figure 2.15

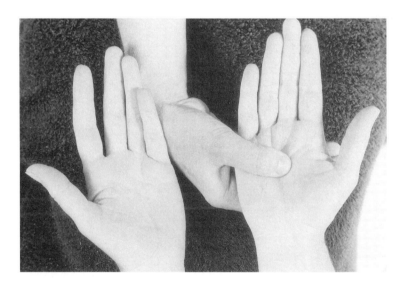

Figure 2.16

Fluid retention

Foot treatment – The lymphatic system protects and cleanses the internal environment of the body with it's fluid. From time to time, for a variety of reasons, the movement of this lymphatic fluid becomes restricted and congested. This presents itself most obviously at the extremities of the hands and feet, when they become swollen, feeling uncomfortable and taut. This can be relieved by using a deep smoothing stroke along the top of the foot in the space between each toe, from the toe towards the ankle. See *Figure 2.17*. This pleasant, comforting stroke can be repeated as much as required. The benefits can be further enhanced by using gravity to assist with the drainage of excess fluid, by having the feet elevated (*Figure 2.18*).

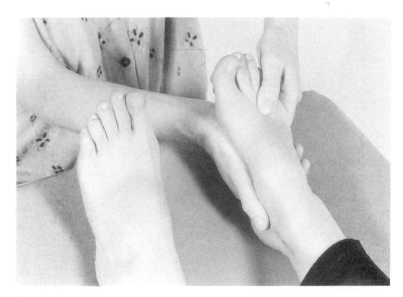

Figure 2.17

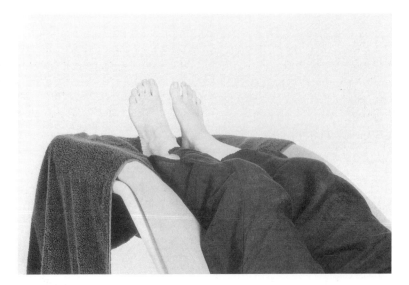

Figure 2.18

Hand treatment – Drainage of the lymphatic system can be encouraged by working the appropriate reflex areas on the back of the hand. See *Figure 2.19*. Use a deep smoothing stroke from the knuckles to the wrist. Again use the assistance of gravity by raising the arm up onto cushions.

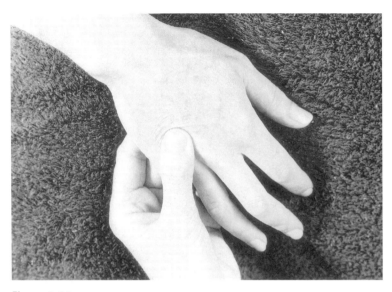

Figure 2.19

Shoulder tension

Foot treatment – In reflexology terms, the shoulders are represented by the large padded area on the sole of the foot at the base of the toes. See *Figure 2.20*. Just as the shoulders are a large muscular part of the body, so the reflex has the same character. Shoulder tension can be eased by using a firm circular thumb pressure over the whole of this area. Both feet should be worked and it can obviously be included within a foot massage sequence.

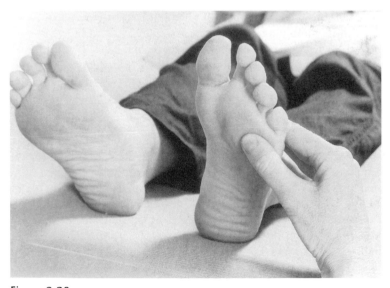

Figure 2.20

Hand treatment – The shoulders are represented in the same way on the hands, being the large area spread over the base of the fingers. See *Figure 2.21*. Interestingly, massaging this area is a familiar movement often used in stressful situations – perhaps as an instinctive reaction to alleviate anxiety?

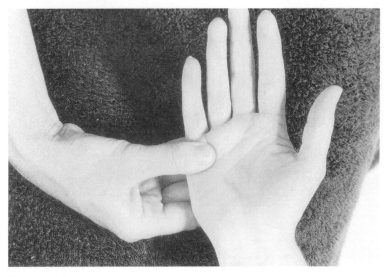

Figure 2.21

Foot care

Once we accept that the state of the body is reflected in the feet, we must also accept that this is a two-way system so, therefore, the state of the feet affects the health of the body. Working with this premise, it is obvious that we should pay attention to how we care for our feet. The bones, ligaments and muscles are arranged in the feet for strength, shock-absorption and load-bearing. The internal intelligence of the body is constantly adjusting to information received via the nerves and the circulation. Our feet not only take care of the active movements of walking and running, but also, they make it possible for us to be balanced and upright. We take most of this for granted but with just a little care our feet,and the whole of our body, can benefit enormously.

Barefoot – Whenever possible, taking the shoes off and walking on an uneven surface is good exercise. Hard, unyielding surfaces, such as concrete, cause strain throughout the body so natural surfaces such as grass or sand are preferable, providing a 'give' to cushion the body. When the feet are without the constraints of shoes, they can spread into a natural pattern and the muscles are fully used.

Badly fitting shoes not only have an effect on the feet themselves, but also on the entire structure of the body, by interfering with its natural balance and alignment. The resulting pressures and restrictions can then go on to affect all the systems of the body.

Circulation of the feet – Effective circulation is essential for the feet and for the overall health of the body.

Deep breathing promotes the movement of fresh blood around the whole of the body, so adopting the breathing techniques described in *Chapter 3 (p.32)* would be very beneficial.

Specifically, breathing in this way can be helpful in reducing the severity and frequency of cramp. This painful condition is caused by the build-up of acidic toxins in the blood, which in turn causes poor muscle function. We eliminate toxins in a variety of ways, either via the kidneys in the form of urine, or via the skin or by breathing. Using deep breathing exercises encourages the elimination of toxins and fresh blood is carried to the tissues

To create a sensation of warmth from the inside out, exercise the feet regularly to create a vigorous blood flow. Even for people who have a sedentary lifestyle, this can be achieved by performing simple exercises, such as rolling the bare feet over a tennis ball, gripping a pencil with the toes or, simply, by wriggling the toes whenever you think about it.

Hydrotherapy for the feet – This simple, economical treatment can be very beneficial for the entire circulation of the body as described in *Chapter 6 (p. 62)* . Simply fill a bath with ankle-deep cold water and walk up and down the bath, lifting the feet clear of the water with each step.

Professional reflexology treatment

There is much that can be achieved through reflexology beyond the self-help approach. It can be used as a complete health care system. There are times when a consultation with a qualified practitioner is needed for various reasons. You may feel that you need the skill and knowledge of a reflexologist alongside your own expert knowledge, in order to give you further support and advice. You may feel that you need to talk about and 'off-load' or share your health concerns. Or you may feel, and it is quite valid, that you want some 'time-out' and to place yourself, literally, in someone else's hands. As well as being a valid form of health care, reflexology sessions are pleasant, enjoyable experiences, being opportunities to feel truly treated.

As already explained, reflexology does not focus on a specific symptom but, instead, aims to achieve a state of balance for the body. More often than not however, it is a symptom that brings someone for a treatment, and, hopefully, these symptoms can be relieved in the process of restoring harmony. Symptoms which can be addressed are many and various, including migraine headaches, digestive problems, circulatory disorders, respiratory conditions, back pain, hormonal imbalances etc.

Reflexology is a powerful tool for promoting relaxation and, as such, it can be extremely beneficial in addressing stress-related conditions.

Reflexology addresses health issues on all levels – physical, emotional and spiritual – and it recognises that these levels have equal status, are intermingled and affect each other continually.

An experienced practitioner will always use a multi-faceted approach by referring to the effect of nutrition, exercise and relaxation on our health. In this way, it may be possible to make appropriate life-styles changes in order to improve our health. Relevant and realistic self-help techniques lead to a continued increase in awareness and confidence for the individual concerned.

As a course of treatment progresses, the recipient may choose to explore the nature of the meaning behind their state of health. It is possible to learn from the 'message' of the current problem, so that it can lead to a positive outcome. This often means working preventatively and also provides an optimistic outlook for future health. This situation may be used to make positive changes for the future. Sometimes it is obvious to see that the manner of the physical symptoms matches the emotional or spiritual state. Sometimes this connection is more hidden than others and a degree of self-reflection and gentle analysis is needed. Often the realisation is enough, in itself, to allow significant improvements to take place and it needs no more attention than that. This increased clarity continues to build on the individual's confidence to trust their self-knowledge.

When not to treat

There are few contraindications to a full reflexology treatment but, occasionally, a practitioner may feel that it is inappropriate. Usually this is when extra stimulus would not be beneficial, for instance with cases of deep vein thrombosis or in the very early stages of pregnancy. It is rare not to be able to treat at all and the more familiar scenario is for experienced practitioners to know when to exercise caution and to use modifications.

3
Yoga

Yoga encompasses an holistic approach to health care by using physical movements (asanas), breathing and relaxation techniques in order to establish a sense of awareness and integration within each person. It has foundations in eastern philosophy which are, nevertheless, relevant to the modern, Western lifestyle; it can help to reduce the inevitable stresses and strains, either physically and/or emotionally.

Yoga asanas work by stretching, strengthening and massaging all structures of the body. For example, a forward bending posture stretches the muscles of the spine and of the legs and also, by compassing the front of the body, it gently massages internal organs.

The practice and study of yoga can be esoteric and mystical if you choose it to be but it also has many practical applications for everyday western life. There is also a myth that you must be flexible before you can practice yoga, in actual fact this is not so, although many people experience an improvement in their flexibility when yoga becomes a regular feature in their lives. It is available for everyone – all ages, all shapes and sizes. Yoga encompasses physical exercises (asanas), breathing and relaxation techniques as well as a philosophy for living; each individual being able to practice whichever of these elements seem relevant at the time. Yoga recognises that people's bodies are like the people – they reflect our state of health, physically and emotionally. Despite popular belief, yoga doesn't always demand a state of calmness – this would be unrealistic and not a true reflection of the rich pattern of life. What it can do, is to make us more aware of how we are actually feeling and of how our physical body affects our emotions and vice versa. This increased awareness often leads to a corresponding increase in confidence and an ability to manage day-to-day situations so that it has very real, practical implications. In this way, each person's yoga becomes their own.

The classical asanas can be adapted to suit each individual and modified for all abilities and needs. Each yoga practice session can also provide a way in which to break the pattern of stress; being a quiet time and an opportunity for self-attention in the midst of busy daily life.

In the West we talk about our hormones and the effect that they have on our emotions and we can all relate to this in the sense of the 'ups and downs' that we feel from time to time. In the oriental sense this may be referred to as an energy system, the presentation of the spirit which makes us the individuals that we are. Yoga aims to restore balance into this system, enabling each person to take from it whatever they need.

This energy, often referred to as 'subtle', is constantly changing. As with all energy, it equates to movement and this movement is life. Yoga aims to put each person, intuitively, in touch with this changing energy in order to maintain health. Many factors can affect us energetically, such as nutrition, climate, exercise, relaxation, our environment, relation-ships, stress levels and so on. All these factors can, at different times in our lives, allow us to feel motivated, energised, fulfilled and nourished or, alternatively, depleted, anxious, depressed and tired. Yoga acknowledges that this is **life** and **human** and it provides a way to increase our awareness of ourselves, so that we can register these feelings and attempt to understand why they are happening.

It is ideal to practice the postures in a calm, focused environment with time which is set aside for this purpose but, often there is real benefit to be gained by isolating certain ones to use as movements during daily life. An ideal approach is to enjoy the actual movement contained within yogic practice – just as children move – with simple pleasure.

Yoga asanas

There are many, many yoga postures, this chapter shows just a few of these with possible modifications to suit individual need and ability. They can be used to maintain fitness and, with variations, to aid recovery after an illness or injury, aiming to prevent a recurrence of the problem. As with any new regime, the initial practice should be one of gentle exploration and all the postures can be refined as experience increases. Commonsense guidelines apply and, if suffering from a medically diagnosed condition, it is advisable to consult your physician. Do not practice immediately after meals.

Triangle pose (Sanskrit: *Trikonasana*)

This standing posture strengthens and tones the large muscles of the spine, legs and shoulders, promotes deep breathing and releases spinal tension.

Method

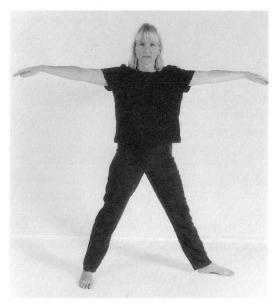

* Stand with the feet wide apart turned to one side. Inhale and extend the arms to shoulder height. See *Figure 3.1*.

* Exhale and tilt slowly sideways towards pointed foot, resting the lower arm on the leg. (The extent of this tilting movement needs to be matched to individual ability.) Extend the upper arm to the ceiling and turn to look towards the hand. Hold while breathing deeply. See *Figure 3.2*. Please note, to achieve optimum benefit in this asana, it is important to maintain a **sideways** position and not to try to increase the movement by leaning forwards.

* Inhale, slowly stand up and repeat to the other side.

Figure 3.1

The shape of this posture allows the body to feel open and extended which encourages the lungs to move to their full capacity on both the inhalation and the exhalation. The nature of the pose is one of confidence and strength, valuable attributes which can be felt during this sequence.

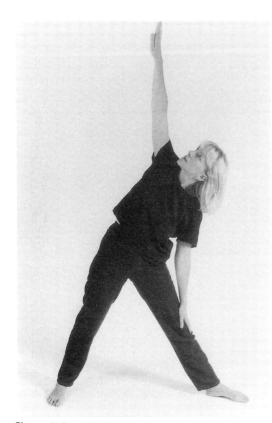

Figure 3.2

Forward bend (*Paschimottanasana*)

This posture flexes the muscles of the upper and lower spine, tones abdominal muscles and gently massages internal organs. The muscles of the legs are also stretched and strengthened.

Method

* Sit on the floor with legs extended, resting the arms on the legs. See *Figure 3.3*.

* Inhale deeply and, on exhalation, relax the upper body forward – moving the hands down as you fold over your legs. See *Figure 3.4*.

* Hold the posture as you breathe deeply, relaxing into the stretch.

* Inhale and return to sitting.

Instead of focusing on how far you can fold towards your legs, this pose can be safely enhanced by being aware of the **length** of your spine, visualising it becoming longer as the position is held.

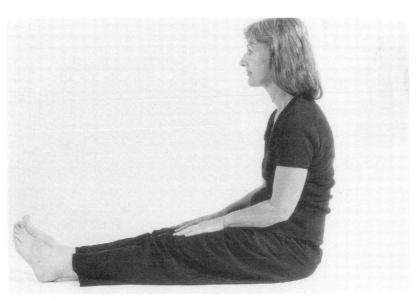

Figure 3.3

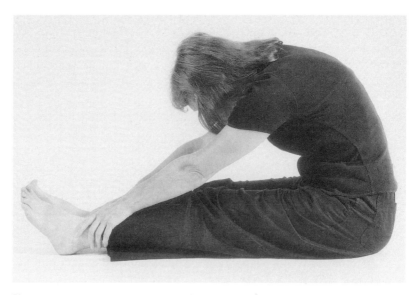

Figure 3.4

Enjoyment and relaxation are also achieved by feeling a sense of release on each exhalation.

As an introduction to this posture or, indeed, at times when a more gentle style is needed, it can be safely modified by bending the legs and placing the arms under the knees. In this way, the upper body is supported and the head and neck can relax over the knees. See *Figure 3.5*.

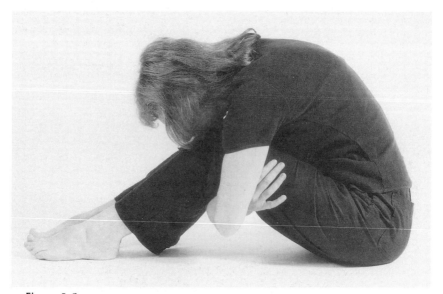

Figure 3.5

Please note, there is also a further variation of this pose in *Chapter 7 (pp. 80–81)*.

In contrast to the forward bend, the **Cobra (*Bhujangasana*)** assists the body with a backward bending movement. It improves flexibility and strength in the lower spine and allows the lungs to expand, facilitating deep breathing. This obviously improves lung function as well as reducing any feelings of stress and anxiety by lowering nervous tension.

Method

* Lie on the floor, face down. Hands are placed palm downwards beneath the shoulders. The chin rests on the floor. See *Figure 3.6*.

* Inhale and raise the head, shoulders and chest from the floor, taking the weight in the hands. The arms remain slightly bent with elbows tucked close to the body. The head looks straight ahead. Breathe deeply and hold the position. Be aware of any possible shoulder tension and attempt to release this on each exhalation. See *Figure 3.7*.

* Exhale and lower the body to the floor slowly. Rest the arms by the side, turn the face to one side and rest, breathing deeply.

* To rest and counter the backward movement of this asana it is helpful then to push up on to the hands and knees and, immediately, to lower down on to the heels with the forehead resting on the bent arms – in the **Child pose**. See *Figure 3.8*.

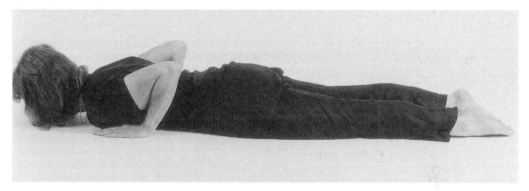

Figure 3.6

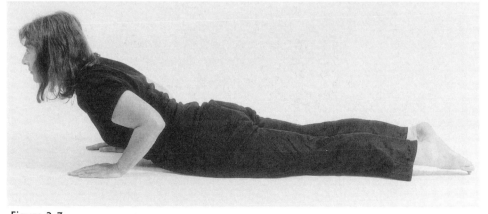

Figure 3.7

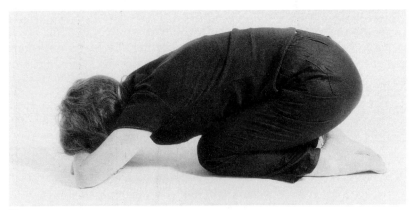

Figure 3.8

The characteristics of the power and strength of the Cobra can often be experienced when maintaining this confident, forward-looking posture. This is then balanced, both physically and emotionally, by resting in the comforting, enclosed posture of the Child. Yoga can represent the duality of our experiences and emotions, acknowledging the validity of all perspectives. At certain periods in our lives, it is possible to relate to some aspects more than others, depending on our circumstances, health and emotional state at that time. For instance, we may feel that we need the benefit of some additional confidence that the Cobra can generate, or perhaps it just expresses how we are feeling and so it feels appropriate. Equally, we may feel that we need the comfort and security that the Child posture provides.

If there is any weakness or injury in the lower back or abdomen, it is advisable to modify the Cobra by resting the forearms on the floor in the **Sphinx** pose. See *Figure 3.9*. This carries the same benefits but in a gentler format. Often the modification is more beneficial because it assists relaxation and allows a more positive sense of success.

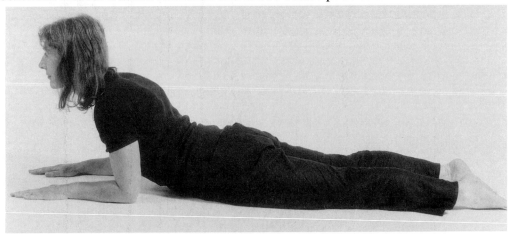

Figure 3.9

Rotation postures in yogic practice are important in that they strengthen the muscles which support the spinal vertebrae. This support helps to maintain a strong, healthy spine and prevents those all-too-familiar back problems experienced with pain and frustration by so many people. Often people report having 'put their back out' while performing a simple, everyday movement. These situations are frequently after a physically or emotionally demanding time, when additional support would be very welcome.

One asana which develops this sense of support is the **Half-spinal twist (*Ardha-Matsyendrasana*)**.

Method

* Sit on the floor with legs extended. Bend the right leg so that the foot rests flat on the floor next to the left knee. Place the right hand on the floor behind for support. Wrap the left arm around the right knee so as to gently compress the leg against the body. See *Figure 3.10*.

* Inhale deeply and, on exhalation, turn to look over the right shoulder. See *Figure 3.11*. Breathe deeply and hold the position.

* Inhale and return to face forward. Repeat to the other side.

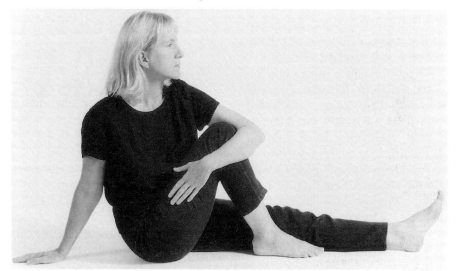

Figure 3.10

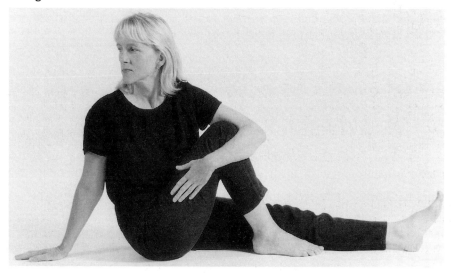

Figure 3.11

In addition to the attention that the muscles of the spine received in this posture, the compression of the abdomen provides a gentle internal massage. This nourishes and benefits the organs of the whole of the pelvic cavity and, specifically, can provide relief for disorders of the digestive system. For further advice on treating disorders of the digestive system, see *Chapter 5* on nutrition.

The awareness in this pose is to feel the strength (not strain) of the muscles extending, in a spiralling motion, from the hips through to the shoulders. As the position is held, with deep breathing to assist with relaxation, a sense of release can be felt physically, and emotionally.

The many rotation postures in yoga can be beneficial in preventing future injuries where there is an established weakness. It is necessary to exercise caution when recovering from a recent injury. A modification of this pose is to sit on a chair and then to rotate gently, using the chair for support. See *Figure 3.12*. Incidentally, this is also particularly beneficial on long train and car journeys.

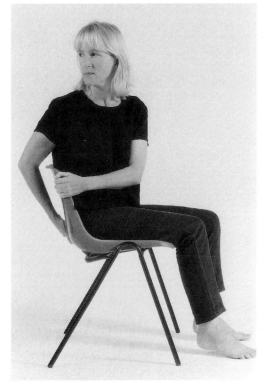

Figure 3.12

The Cat (*Marjaraiasana*)

This posture enhances the flexibility of the spine and massages the whole of the pelvic region. It is particularly beneficial for women, assisting with relief for menstrual disorders. It has special relevance during pregnancy (*Chapter 7*).

Method

* Kneel on the floor on hands and knees. Inhale and gently look up, feeling a slight hollow of the spine. See *Figure 3.13*.

* Exhale, look down towards the knees, forming an arch of the spine. Relax the head and neck. See *Figure 3.14*.

* Repeat as often as you wish, always synchronising the movement with the breath.

It enhances this posture to focus on the rhythm of the spinal movement, being aware of the flexibility along the vertebrae. In addition, if the abdominal muscles are contracted on each exhalation, this provides a gentle internal massage and can assist greatly with conditions of the digestive system.

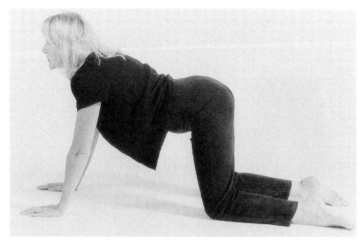

Figure 3.13

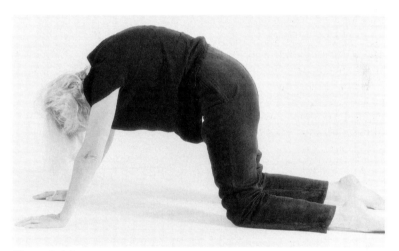

Figure 3.14

Shoulderstand (*Sarvangasana*)

The sanskrit name means literally 'all parts pose' indicating the benefits that the entire body can receive from this posture. Human beings spend a large part of each day standing and walking with resulting pressure and compression on the structures and organs of the lower body. This can contribute to, among others, digestive problems, impaired circulation, menstrual disorders and back pain. It can be extremely beneficial to reverse these effects of gravity by inverting the body. The concept of upside-down postures in yoga is often daunting but realistic adaptations can mean that this can be achieved for the majority of people.

The Shoulderstand is one way to achieve this inversion.

Method

* Lie on your back on the floor. Bend your legs, placing your feet flat on the floor, resting arms by your side. See *Figure 3.15*.

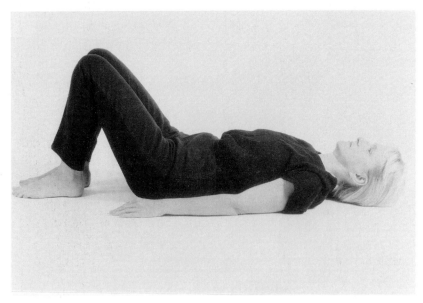

Figure 3.15

* Inhale, raising the legs, supporting your body with hands on hips. See *Figure 3.16*. This is the half-shoulderstand and is a complete posture in itself. If you wish to continue with the full posture continue with the next step.

* Raise the legs straight in the air, 'walking' the hands down the spine for support. See *Figure 3.17*. Breathe deeply and relax the legs while holding the posture.

* To come down, lower the knees to the head, rest the hands down to the floor and tuck the chin in to the chest while rolling the spine down to the floor. See *Figure 3.18*.

* Rest, taking at least three deep breaths into the chest area to counter any compression that may have been experienced .

In addition to the benefits already mentioned, this posture strengthens the muscles of the spine and abdomen and develops our sense of balance. It is enhanced by breathing deeply, allowing the entire length of the legs to feel relaxed and appreciating the relief from weight-bearing to the lower half on the body – feeling this as a relief from pressure – in all its forms.

A degree of caution and common sense needs to be exercised with this posture, especially if there is any weakness to the muscles of the spine and abdomen. It requires a degree of strength and control and it may be appropriate when yogic practice is relatively new, or when a less strenuous approach is indicated, to modify this posture. This adaptation of the classical asanas is part of the richness and pleasure of yoga, there is always an element of progression, giving each person a further sense of achievement. It is never success or failure, or better or worse but instead it acknowledges the individuality of people, so that each of us can practice yoga in a way that is appropriate to us at that moment in time.

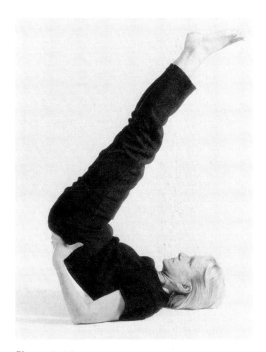

Figure 3.16

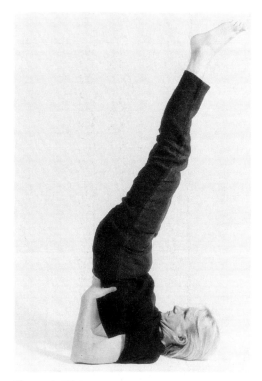

Figure 3.17

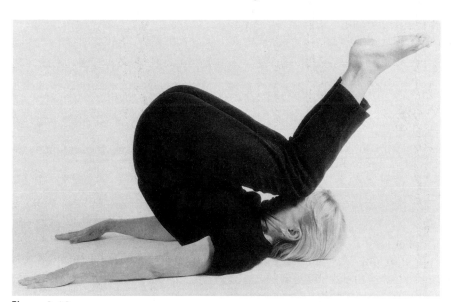

Figure 3.18

A modification of Shoulderstand is to use the floor and wall as support. See *Figure 3.19*. This is extremely relaxing and it equals the full extension of the posture in its ability to relieve weight and pressure from the supporting structures and organs of the body. It can be used to great effect to relieve some of the discomfort during pregnancy (*Chapter 7*), and for any conditions where relief from pressure is indicated, for example, painful menstruation or

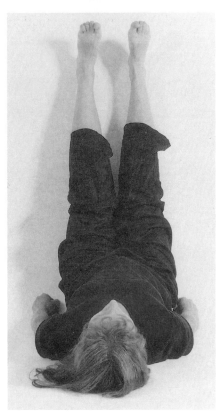

Figure 3.19

disorders of the digestive system (see *Chapter 5*).

All yoga is best learnt under the guidance of a qualified teacher, this can be either in a class situation or in a one-to-one consultation. There is a true richness and enjoyment with all aspects of the discipline that can be used and adapted to suit each individual, so that each person can make each session their own yoga.

Breathing

There are many breathing techniques which can be included in the practice of yoga, all with specific benefits. The fundamental principle is that, in order to obtain maximum benefit from our breathing, it is important to use the whole of the structure of the breathing mechanism, ie. the lungs.

The action of breathing is often taken for granted and it is easy to become lazy about it.

The most basic, and most beneficial, breathing technique is the 'three-part' breath; this uses the whole of the lungs with advantages for the entire body, mind and spirit.

Three-part breath

This is ideal to be practised lying down for additional relaxation benefit. However, in time, as it becomes more familiar and instinctive, it is possible to use this technique to defuse stressful situations wherever you may be, to boost energy levels when needed or, simply to be aware of efficient, effective breathing. Young children breathe in this way automatically and, therefore, for adults, it is often enjoyable to discover this free movement again.

Method

* Lie on the floor, legs bent. See *Figure 3.20*. Rest your hands on your belly. As you breathe in, visualise taking your breath into the space beneath your hands, allowing your belly to gently rise. Exhale and feel the muscles relax. Repeat for three breaths.

* Move your hands to rest on the rib cage. See *Figure 3.21*. Again breathe into this space, feel the expansion of the ribs as your hands are gently pushed out. Exhale and follow the movement of the ribs, gently squeezing them to complete the exhalation. Repeat for three breaths.

* Now move the hands to rest on your collar bones. See *Figure 3.22*. Breathe into this space – there will just be a slight movement now. Again feel the relaxation as you exhale. Repeat for three breaths.

* For the complete breath, these three stages are combined. You may wish to continue using your hands for guidance initially. Aim for a smooth transition from one stage to another and a steady, even expansion throughout the full area.

* There is a distinction between the nature of the inhalation and the exhalation. The inhalation is energetic and vital whereas the exhalation has a sense of release and ease.

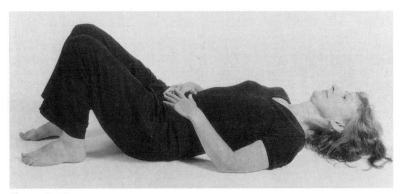

Figure 3.20

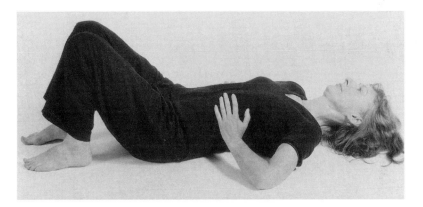

Figure 3.21

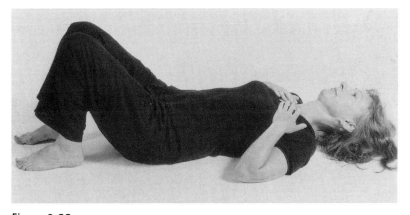

Figure 3.22

Efficient, effective breathing can benefit all the systems of the body:

Soothes the nerves – In stressful situations, the body needs to breathe rapidly with energy being supplied to the structures of the body that are needed for action. The benefit of deep breathing exercises is that these stress responses are reversed; this has a calming effect on the entire nervous system and on the messages that it transmits throughout the mind and body. In addition to promoting relaxation, as the nervous system is soothed and eased, this gives a valuable method of pain control.

Improve digestive function – The movement generated with breathing exercises, namely that of the diaphragm, provides a massage for the internal organs of the digestive system.

Ventilate the lungs – The lungs themselves are completely ventilated and used to maximum capacity. Fresh air is used to 'air' every corner of the lungs so that they remain healthy.

Maximum circulation – There is an analogy here where the breath is used as 'fuel' to light the 'fire', ie. the energy and nourishment of the body. In a sense adequate oxygenation leads to efficient combustion of fuel. Correct breathing means that the body will receive optimum benefit from its nourishment and circulation so that every system of the body will benefit. The resulting improved circulation means that fresh, healthy blood takes nourishment around the entire body.

De-tox the whole body – There is currently much advice in the media on the importance of the many and varied ways to 'de-tox' the body. This process can be encouraged simply, effectively and economically, by the introduction of adequate breathing techniques. As a system, the body has several ways in which it removes unwanted material and strives to maintain a healthy, clean environment. This elimination of toxins is via the intestines, the kidneys, the skin and the breath. Deep, effective breathing allows oxygenation to 'burn up' harmful acidic wastes. This relieves the burden on the other organs of elimination; it 'shares the load'. Attention to breathing exercises can be especially helpful when there is a specific need to de-tox, for instance, if taking any form of medication, or after over-indulging with food or drink. There are various ways that the body shows evidence of being over-loaded with toxins, these include; aches and pains in the joints, skin conditions, tiredness, headaches, digestive disorders or respiratory conditions. Effective breathing would be a beneficial addition to the treatment of these conditions, supported by modifications to eating habits (see advice given *Chapter 5, p. 44*).

It is easy to see how, on all levels, a simple breathing technique can have a positive effect. It has the added bonus of being very economical and totally portable! It can become a useful 'tool' to draw on when needed, wherever you are, at the office desk, in the bus queue or when doing the washing-up.

Importance of correct posture with breathing

One simple, quick way to improve breathing capacity is to give attention to our posture. Allowing the back muscles to slouch and the shoulders to become rounded means that the physical capacity of the lungs is compromised, in other words, there is less space to breathe into. This can be easily remedied, whenever you think about it, whether you are sitting or standing, by checking:

- that you are sitting/standing tall through the entire length of your spine
- that your shoulders are wide open and relaxed.

Some breathing exercises use a more concentrated degree of control than others, these can be especially helpful as part of a programme to reduce stress and tension. They introduce a greater feeling of control and focus, becoming almost like a meditation process. It is possible to be so involved in the process that external concerns and anxieties are excluded. One such method is to use counting to direct the breathing.

'Counting' breathing technique

Method

* Breathe in, using the whole of the lungs as described in the 'three-part breathing' technique. While inhaling count silently to yourself, initially count slowly to four.

* Breathe out fully. The exhalation is longer than the inhalation, so now count up to eight.

* Continue in this way for three breaths. Ensure that each inhalation and exhalation is exercised to the full extent. The inhalation feeling dynamic and energised, while the exhalation feels steady and controlled. This reinforces the duality of yogic practice with both power and energy existing alongside a sense of ease and relaxation.

* Be aware of the pauses between the in and the out-breath. After the next inhalation, hold the breath as you count to two. Breathe out, and then suspend the breath as you count to two. Repeat each 'round' of breathing three times, maintaining this rhythm of 4–2–8–2.

* With increased practice, the numbers can be increased but always maintain the same ratio. For example, it could be 8–4–16–4.

Focused attention on breathing gives us a way to be aware of the movement and function of the body: to observe it with wonder, at the same time as participating with both pleasure and confidence.

4

Relaxation and rest

The benefits of relaxation and rest cannot be underestimated, however, generally speaking, no time is allowed for either in modern western life. If these can be regarded as opportunities to restore energy back into a busy life then they would seem to be essential and for everyone's benefit, for the individual concerned and for everyone that he/she comes into contact with.

Visualisation and meditation are also ways to spend quiet, reflective time in order to restore yourself physically, emotionally and spiritually. Each of these activities can be adapted to suit individual need, preference and lifestyle so that they become a comfortable, familiar part of life.

Relaxation

We all need an element of stress in our lives providing us with stimulus and motivation. Our bodies are designed to cope with stress in the short term and this can be seen as a positive state. Unfortunately, in the modern world stress is constant, long term and very negative. Relaxation provides a way of breaking this inappropriate stress pattern. The benefits exist on all levels of being – physical, emotional and spiritual.

This is particularly relevant when we consider the high percentage of all illness which is now recognised as having a root cause in stress. This includes headaches, back pain, heart conditions, high blood pressure, respiratory and digestive disorders, skin conditions and hormonal imbalances. We can all relate to that feeling of being drained emotionally when under pressure and needing an opportunity to stand back from situations in order to see events more clearly. Relaxation, in whatever form, can provide this necessary time to look at situations in perspective, to be able to assess and review and to look ahead.

Relaxation can take many forms, some more structured than others, but it is important to emphasise that it should always feel appropriate to one's lifestyle and personality. It can be achieved by retrieving a favourite activity that has been 'squeezed out' because of a busy life, eg. walking, cycling, fishing etc. Or perhaps it is an opportunity to pursue a new hobby, or something that you have been meaning to get around to but have just not managed to.

It may be that you build into your daily routine just ten minutes of exclusive time for yourself. Perhaps this is in the morning so that you can plan the day ahead, to prioritise and focus on the tasks to come. Or it could be at the end of the day, giving an opportunity to review the successes, and failures, so that you can 'draw a line under' that part of your life, clear your mind and go from work mode into family mode. This can be a way to avoid the scenario of different factions of life becoming fused together with a feeling of not doing any of them well. With these few moments, it is possible to be able to apply oneself successfully to each role. You will feel more satisfied and those around you will benefit from your focused attention.

Relaxation can be active or otherwise, sociable or solitary – as long as it feels that this is your exclusive time. Maybe you go for a walk or a run, or just sit quietly in the garden or the park. It is an opportunity to focus on yourself and to be attentive to your own needs. It may require some effort and adjustments to the normal routine but that is the challenge.

There are structured relaxation techniques which are quiet and focused with obvious benefits. Some people relate to this approach more than others.

Relaxation techniques

* The environment is ideally quiet, warm and free from distractions.

* Lie down, making sure you are warm and comfortable. Feel supported by the floor. Gently close your eyes.

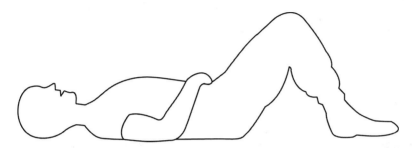

* Then, take a few moments to concentrate on breathing, allowing it to become slow and steady, using the lungs to their extent (as described in *Chapter 3, p.32*: the 'three part-breath'). This deep breathing, practised with awareness supports the relaxation process. No conscious movement, except for this breathing, is required now. It is an opportunity for the nervous system to rest, being still and quiet. When responding to a stressful situation, necessary physical changes take place in the human body, one of these being that breathing becomes rapid and shallow. By allowing the breath to become slow and steady, the internal 'messages' to the body are relaying a state of relaxation. Be conscious of the movement that is created as you breathe; the steady, even expansion on the inhalation and the sense of softening and ease on the exhalation.

* Take this awareness of your breath throughout your body, for example, feel that the inhalation can be directed down to your feet and that it is warming and nourishing, sending vital energy down your ankles, feet and toes. On the exhalation, visualise any tension or discomfort gently drifting away. Practice this exercise up through your body, to each part in turn – legs, hips, back, belly, chest, hands, arms, shoulders, neck, back of the head, face, forehead – until all of you begins to feel at ease and relaxed. If any area needs special attention then return to it and repeat the process, directing the breath and energy there and then releasing the tension/discomfort.

* Allow your mind, treating it as just another part of you, to be equally still and calm. Let any thoughts drift in, and, just as freely, drift away again – giving them no particular attention. Be patient with yourself, just allow these thoughts to drift away. This is often the most challenging part of any relaxation session, so be kind to yourself, don't struggle with this and give yourself lots of time. Remember that some days will be easier than others, but whatever shape the relaxation takes will be beneficial to you; it will be your time, exclusively for you. Continue to use your breathing, feel the inhalation bringing energy and a sensation of clarity. On the exhalation, allow your mind to feel calm and still. Just as you allow physical tension to be released with the exhalation, you can also

for these few moments, let go of anxieties and concerns. Often people find that when they return to these thoughts, they are able to look at them more clearly, having a sense of perspective. It may be helpful to see, in your mind's eye, words such as 'clear', 'calm' and 'still'. Practice the idea of being pleasantly, confidently detached – neither asleep, nor awake.

* When you end the session, give yourself time to adjust and prepare to be alert again. First of all, consciously connect back with your breathing again, allowing it to adjust to a normal rate. Begin to move and stretch, the smallest muscles first of all – fingers, toes and face. Then increase the movement more and more, as you feel ready. Slowly open your eyes. Sit up in your own time. It is helpful to have a few moments to adjust after the relaxation .

* In just a short time, perhaps even ten minutes, relaxation can create a feeling of being restored and refreshed. This constructive time reaps rewards for the rest of the day – and it is enjoyable!

Visualisation

Visualisation is an enormously enriching activity and merely an extension of – you could perhaps say, a training of – something that we all engage in from time to time, ie. day-dreaming. This is a pleasant way to 'step-out' from everyday life for a few moments, although it may not always be appropriate. Human beings are capable of holding a picture in the mind's eye and this can be used very positively.

Visualisation is a way of removing all the 'clutter' from the mind by focusing on one specific image and on the details associated with that image. If/when the mind begins to wander away from the image, gently bring it back again. Using this gentle discipline, all the busy thoughts are removed and the mind is given the opportunity to become calm. It may be that you choose to concentrate on an object, for instance, a tree and this may be an imaginary one or a favourite real one. The focus would then be on the visual beauty of the tree, the colour, size, light, movement and shape of it. You could sit quietly in the shade of the tree and be focused on it. Or, perhaps you have a memory of a special tree and you could return to that, no matter how far away you are physically.

Another example would be to take yourself, in your mind's eye, to a place which has special significance for you, somewhere where you felt particularly safe, calm and happy. If this is the case, you can focus on all the sights, sounds and sensations that you associate with that place.

By allowing our senses to become more receptive to the wonder and beauty of the world around us, we respond by becoming more relaxed and more aware. There are any number of structured visualisations which guide the mind through a scene, allowing it to form its own impressions guided by the senses. An example of one would be:

Guided visualisation

* For a few moments, settle into the session by concentrating on your breathing. Practice your, now familiar, deep breathing exercises.

* Imagine yourself walking by the side of a river. This may be a real place, or an imaginary one. It is a quiet, warm, sunny day.

* **See**, in your mind's eye, a clear blue sky. The water in the river is clear and fresh, with the sun shining and sparkling on its surface. You can see around you a variety of trees and flowers and all their colours, some close by you are vivid and sharp and others, further away, are merged together.

* **Hear** the birds singing around you. You can hear the sound of the running water.

* You can **feel** the texture of the ground underneath your feet. How does this feel?

* You can **smell** flowers, the earth and fresh air.

* After a few moments you can rest under the shade of a tree and drink from the clear, clean water of the river. This **tastes** refreshing and reviving. You have time to rest here.

* When you are ready, you walk back along the river returning to the place where you started.

* Give yourself time to return to everyday life. Consciously connect to your breathing again and become aware of your surroundings, where you are touching the floor and where you are in the room. You return to day-to-day activity again but hold on to the benefits of this session. Register how you feel, acknowledge the freshness in your mind.

Visualisation is often used to support the body's ability to heal itself. This is a completely subjective, personal exercise with each individual choosing the image that comes into their own mind and which is appropriate to them. For example, cancer sufferers often relate visualising damaged cells becoming clear, vibrant and well or they imagine these cells leaving their body and being replaced by strong, healthy ones. This isn't a destructive, attacking process but instead it recognises that every part of that person is a vital, necessary, integral part of them. Rather than being negative, it allows attention and care to be directed to an area that needs it. It works with the body rather than against it. This approach provides psychological support and comfort at a vital time and it enables the person to feel involved in their own health. It supports whatever care regime each individual has elected to use, whether this be complementary or allopathic.

As with a structured relaxation session, for visualisation you should aim to set aside a time when you can be free from interruptions and to be in a place which is conducive to such a quiet activity. This is a valuable process in itself, establishing quality, attentive time.

Meditation

Relaxation encourages a positive, detached observation of the body. Visualisation uses imagery to relax and restore energy in a detailed, structured manner. Meditation, on the other hand, gives the mind freedom to dwell on a concept with a sense of self-control. It provides internal focus giving the mind a freer rein to pursue a theme, a thought. It can promote a great sense of slowing down, becoming still within oneself. The ideal environment is in a quiet place but, once practised, it can be a valuable technique to draw on in the most unlikely places when needed or just whenever the opportunity arises. Perhaps whenever you have a 'gift' of some unexpected time, for example, when waiting at the hairdressers or, to turn a negative situation into a positive one, when the train is late. When applied to specific issues, meditation can provide solutions, allowing decisions to be made with a sense of 'stepping back', being able to view a situation and to think things through. It certainly gives a feeling of taking time out of a busy world and, thus, 'recharging', strengthening and reducing stress levels. Your meditation can last for quite long periods of time in a room devoted to that purpose or just for a few moments – it is very adaptable to need and, more importantly, to available time. In fact, meditation could be said to be any quiet, reflective, contemplative time. In this wider sense, it might then be a walk in the country, an afternoon's gardening or sitting in the local park.

It may be that you choose to meditate on a personal issue, an area of your life that you feel needs some attention and clarity. This may be something that you need to make a decision about or something that you need to be clearer about in your own mind. It is an opportunity to muse, to ponder, to assess, to reappraise situations. Or you could decide to concentrate on a wider theme, perhaps a topic that interests you in the world in general. Or, you may want to look at a specific object and, to quote from the previous example, this could be your **favourite tree**. This could be in your mind's eye or you could be lucky enough to be sitting under the tree itself. Ideally it is a conducive environment, either in reality or reproduced in mind from your memory. Now, as well as being aware of all the physical attributes of the said tree, you can allow your mind to explore deeper, less tangible elements. For instance:

- consider its history and what it may have been witness to
- where does it get its energy from?
- what does it give back to the world?
- where do its roots go?

These thoughts may then lead you to consider issues such as; are your roots solid and, whatever the answer, would you like to change this? Where do you get your energy and nourishment from? Is this adequate? These are just ideas, but see where your mind takes you. Allow it to roam. Say thank-you to the tree.

Another example would be, when you have a few quiet moments, to recall, in your mind's eye, the image of a **bird flying freely in the sky**. You may have a memory that is especially poignant for one reason or another:

- as you begin to picture the image of the bird in your mind, be aware of your breathing becoming slower and steadier. The Sanskrit word for bird is *Hamsa* and this can be used to enhance the tranquillity of the exercise. As you inhale, say to yourself 'Ham', and as you exhale with a sigh, say to yourself 'sa'. Repeat six times.
- now focus on the detail of the bird. Its size, colour and shape. How do its wings move? Is it hovering or flying to a certain place?
- be aware of the colour of the sky. Are there any clouds?
- what noises can you hear?
- what emotions can you recall?
- consider the image of the free flight. What does this symbol of freedom mean to you? What is its relevance to your life just now? Are you as free as you would like to be? If not, can you change that? If you cannot change it, escape to images like this to support and sustain you until you can.
- does this exercise comfort you? Does it inspire you?
- allow your mind to roam where it wants to take you
- initially you could practice this exercise for ten minutes. Then, when you feel ready, you can extend this to twenty, and then thirty, minutes.

After any meditation exercise, allow yourself a few minutes to adjust to the everyday world again. Feel restored, knowing that you can repeat the process as and when required.

When you begin to play with meditation, you may be surprised how it finds its way into your daily routine. It can be used to relieve the tedium and monotony of boring chores, the rhythm of the repetitive task providing an opportunity for the mind to wander.

The spontaneity of meditation can be amazing. When you find yourself in a beautiful place, take time to savour as many details as you can. Then close your eyes and place all of these in your memory. They can then be recalled at a later date when you choose to do so. Not only the visual images, but also the emotions and feelings engendered can be relived. Truly the moment can be captured. The physical and emotional aspects become one entity as sensations are relived. The beauty is in the simplicity; it is always with you, no matter where you are.

Sometimes the results of these contemplative times can be illuminating. The experience will, at least, be enriching and rewarding, providing a few quiet moments to feel replenished and restored. It is a time just to appreciate being still and quiet. Like all new regimes, you may need to be patient with yourself and learn to acquire the skill. Be assured, if it is an effort, that the results are well worth it.

Rest

While relaxation, visualisation and meditation all direct and allow the body and mind to take it easy, there is a very great deal to be said for good, old-fashioned rest. In order for any health care changes to be truly effective they should be accompanied by adequate rest.

Resting is given even less regard in modern daily life than relaxation and is often even seen as a sign of weakness; the implication is that if you need to rest it must be because of being unable to cope with demands. However, when considered within the context of an individual's life at any one time, it can be seen as eminently sensible and, quite obviously, essential. If, for instance, someone is not sleeping well, or just naturally sleeps for only a short time or has irregular working patterns then a daily rest would seem completely relevant. Or, if the normal routine is to wake early and go to bed late, then it would seem apparent to take some time to replenish energy in the middle of the day. After a strenuous working schedule, it would seem to be not only appropriate, but also essential, to take a break before the next demanding period and, in this way, to prevent 'burn-out' and to maintain efficiency for the future. It can also have great restorative powers when energy levels are low after a period of illness. The expectations and pace of modern society do not, unfortunately, allow the necessary time for vital convalescence.

It is difficult to integrate into the modern western pace of life but perhaps that makes it even more valuable and appropriate? Ultimately, it doesn't need to be justified – it is quite simply a time to look after yourself as you deserve.

There are many ways in which to achieve a resting schedule and it will depend on lifestyle, commitments and personal choice which you feel is appropriate. Here are some ideas:

∗ A short (thirty minutes?) daily rest at the time in the day when you feel your energy levels 'dip'. This can be particularly useful when your night time sleeping pattern is disturbed for some reason or other. You could be lying down or in a comfy seat with your feet resting up on a stool. You don't need to be asleep, you could be still and quiet with your own thoughts, or you could be reading – whatever will allow and encourage you to rest.

* A more structured approach may be necessary when feeling stressed or during a period of illness. The irony here is that if you are the sort of person who really needs to do this, then you will be the sort of person who will find it most difficult. The challenge of this may be to allocate a rest-time which is sacrosanct, respected by yourself and those around you. Often it helps to have one special place where you feel peaceful and tranquil. If you have the correct environment, this makes the statement for yourself and for people around you too, that this is your rest time and you are not to be disturbed. Create a situation so that this is a truly enjoyable, positive experience and one that can be looked forward to with anticipation. If you need to justify it, and you probably will, see it as a **treat** and one that is well-deserved.

* It may be a case of 'putting your feet up' at the end of a busy day. Literally put your feet up on a stool – and **don't move**! Even if this is for just a short time, you will have replenished your stock of energy and your whole self can breathe a sigh of relief.

* It is often said 'oh, give it a rest' – meaning we want something to **stop**. A great deal of imagination and inspiration is needed to deal with an area of our lives that is causing us to be stressed or irritated. Give yourself a short, quiet reflective time in which to identify the problem. Often it is worthy of some considered thought to see if this can be eliminated, or at least, modified in some way. If this involves other people, perhaps you need to be assertive, or, at least, very diplomatic. Or perhaps there is a practical solution, for instance, you unplug the telephone for a day. At crucial times, it may be necessary to set aside a day – or even two – to be allocated for total rest. For busy people, and ironically, this only applies to busy people, this will require considerable preparation, making arrangements and notifying people around you but the rewards can be enormous. It is a case of creating a situation in which you can rest physically and emotionally – away from the demands of the outside world. See it as a way of replenishing your reserves. So don't dismiss this notion totally; if you really need it, then it is possible and it will be well worth it.

* In a steady, consistent way, you can feel rejuvenated by the discipline of going to bed early. The old wive's tale of the sleep hours before midnight being worth double those of after midnight seems to be pertinent here. This is because we naturally begin to replenish and restore at this time of the day and this process is more efficient when we are asleep.

* Another maxim 'a change is as good as a rest' is also relevant. There is much to be said for a change of routine, scenery, environment or, perhaps, company. A holiday is the obvious – and enjoyable – answer, giving an opportunity to 'recharge the batteries'. It need not be adventurous, expensive or lengthy, in fact there is real value to be had from taking regular, short breaks.

* One way to provide yourself with internal rest is to reduce the amount of work that your body has to do by eating less. This need not be anything as drastic as a fast which may seem quite alien and would certainly need guidance and supervision. This level of rest can be achieved by simply reducing the amount of food intake, by eating in a kinder, less robust way for a short time. It would be entirely appropriate to accompany this with a time when you can be physically resting too. To assist this it would be helpful, not only to eat less but also to eat fewer of those foods which are more difficult to digest, ie. concentrated proteins (*Chapter 5*). This is certainly true during periods of, and recovering from, illness. Obviously, at these times the body needs quality foods to

support the process of repair and recovery, but not food which is going to take vital energy away in order to be adequately digested. Quality, light, easily digested foods include fresh fruit, salads and vegetables (organic if possible), soup and fish.

* Complementary health care can be supportive to this regime. When receiving a treatment, for example massage or reflexology, you allow yourself, you give yourself permission, to rest for at least the time of the consultation when you are attended to and cared for. Hopefully, the value of this will be so evident that it can then 'spill over' into some other time in your life.

It will depend on how needy you are at certain life stages which option, if any, appeals, and which you feel you can achieve. Or you may have your own ideas. It may not be easy, but if the notion of taking a rest sounds remotely attractive to you, then it probably means that you need to do it. Like all challenges, if successfully faced then it will be rewarding and worthwhile. It can be seen as an investment and, like all investments, it is an opportunity to lay down stores, reserves for the future. Always remember – you have earned it.

5

Nutrition

Enjoyable nutrition

We all enjoy a tremendous variety and availability of food in the western world but this brings its own problems, mainly one of over-consumption. As the huge food industry continues to strive to meet ever-increasing demand, food production processes bring further anxieties. Genuine concerns about food issues are reflected in the high profile that nutrition enjoys within the media. This media attention is often contradictory as it continues to present the 'very latest' eating regimes which are subject to fashion, and guidelines on how and what to eat which are often impractical, unrealistic and add to the overall pattern of anxiety. In the light of this, it would be easy to regard any information relating to eating and food generally as confusing, restricting, guilt-laden and, in fact, that the whole subject is rather disagreeable. All this presents a dilemma in that our first experience of food, ie. being fed by our mothers was a pleasant one and, instinctively, we strive to repeat this. We want to enjoy, not just the food itself, but also the **experience** of eating. This chapter aims to show how it is possible to achieve this and, also, to eat food which can provide the necessary nutrients to maintain and, when required, to assist with restoring health.

How and what we eat is a fundamental way to care for ourselves. There are times when people wish to change or adapt their eating habits, this can be either to address specific issues or, simply, because they feel that there is room for improvement. Typically, this is when contact with a professional is advisable. In a consultation, a unique nutritional profile would be planned, taking into account lifestyle, health issues and personality. This can be refined and adapted as necessary at any subsequent sessions. The consultation environment acting here as a 'resource centre', enabling each person to manage their own nutritional status with confidence and awareness.

Relationship with food

We all have a unique relationship with the food that we eat. This is dependent on a variety of factors, including childhood memories associated with food and eating, lifestyle, cultural background, daily routine, age, occupation and overall state of health, both physical and emotional. The unique nature of this relationship is shown in the way that each of us decides how, what and when to eat. We don't necessarily have to change this but just to be aware of it is often helpful. For instance, do you eat when you are worried? Or perhaps you can't eat when you feel like that? Or do you eat more when you are happy or when you are sad? Do you eat more or less when you are missing someone? Then you could ask yourself, **what** do you eat when you feel these emotions? Like all worthwhile relationships, it is not one to be taken for granted. It is important to have an understanding of it, to see how it can be improved on and, again, like all good relationships, it is not static. How and what we eat affects, and is affected by, everything else that is going on in our lives at any one time. There is no one perfect way to eat because, thankfully, we are all diverse and unique.

This is where the confusion surrounding nutritional issues arises; to look for a definitive guide to eating is an impossible task. But it is this same fact that makes nutrition so fascinating and challenging. We can, each of us, **choose** how to nourish ourselves, to suit personality, lifestyle, level of activity and health. This choice is not written in tablets of stone, we are all dynamic, energetic beings and thankfully the way in which we eat reflects this. As our lives change, so our way of eating changes. We may plan a set of guidelines which suits perfectly but, reassuringly, we can deviate from it at times, for the sake of variety and interest and to prove that we are human. It shouldn't be, as dietary guidelines often are, a source of resentment or guilt. Eating, again from our earliest memories, is meant to be a pleasurable, sociable activity.

'Conscious eating'

Continuing the theme of not taking the food that we eat for granted, we can strive to be **aware** of what we are eating. In other words, to avoid the scenario of 'just eating for the sake of it' or of getting to the end of a meal and then realising you haven't actually consciously **tasted** anything. With this in mind it is worth considering some questions:

- is this food attractive to me? Does it look interesting and colourful?
- am I enjoying this meal?
- do I want to eat this food?
- does the food smell good to me?
- am I actually hungry?

We talk about 'savouring' food, interestingly the word 'savour' can mean to taste or to appreciate and enjoy. Perhaps we can also ask, 'do I savour each mouthful?' By answering these sorts of questions, we can become **conscious** and aware about our food and begin to think about **why** and **how** we eat. This doesn't need to be as clinical as it may seem; you may be aware that the reason you are eating something is because it is a treat.

Positive attitude to nutrition

Any conversations centred around the word 'diet' have come to be synonymous with weight loss and the inevitable associations of deprivation and denial. This illustrates the fact that the major nutritionally-related health problems in the West are associated with over-consumption; it is a fact that we all eat more than we need. However, when we talk about our diet, we really need to refer to all aspects of food intake not just the quantity but also the quality. In addition, when we consider how we each relate to food, how we find a way of eating to suit each one of us, then it becomes a much more vibrant, enthusiastic proposition. To develop a more positive outlook to the subject of nutrition, food becomes not just fuel but how we look after ourselves, how we sustain energy and how we protect ourselves in order to stay healthy. Nutrition also has a pro-active role to play during and after periods of illness, in that it is fundamental in helping the body to repair and restore itself. We are all familiar with how foods rich in vitamin C can defend us from the common cold, but there is now much evidence to show how diet can be used to fight illnesses such as heart disease, asthma and cancer. The German physician, Max Gerson published a book in 1958 entitled *A Cancer Therapy: Results of Fifty Cases*. In this, he outlines his raw food regime which he claims enables patients to fight and destroy cancer cells by stimulating the body's own defence mechanism, the lymphatic system (Kenton, 1995).

How we eat is the ultimate in self-help, a statement about how we choose to care for ourselves. While changes to eating habits almost always present a challenge, it is possible to plan a way of eating that matches individual lifestyle and taste, this then becomes both more attractive and more sustainable.

The importance of whole food

As previously mentioned, advice concerning food issues can seem conflicting and confusing but this can easily be clarified by adopting the common-sense approach that the most nutritious is **whole food**, ie. food which is as nature intended it to be and which has received as little intervention as possible. This is the one consistent fact within all dietary advice, whatever the rationale and reason behind it. This guideline for 'first principle' food means that the goodness, nutritional value, the energy has not been diminished by any treatment, manufacturing or storage process. There is increased concern, both for ourselves and for the environment, centred around food production methods such as the use of organo-phosphates and genetically modified foods (Blythman, 1996). There are valid anxieties concerning the rearing of livestock which has been adapted to meet the needs of the ever-increasing demand of the food industry. The effects of this intervention may not be proven for several decades, however we see examples for ourselves, for instance the BSE epidemic and the effect of certain chemical additives on the health of children. The ultimate example of an ideal food is to be able to pick an orange from a tree and to eat it while it is still warm from the sunshine. The energy is still in the fruit. We can try to replicate this as much as possible, by buying fresh, organic produce or better still, by growing our own. The added bonus is that it tastes better too.

The manner of eating

As well as considering **what** to eat , there is much to be said for paying attention to **how** we eat. The Eastern philosophy on this states that if you eat when you are angry, hurried or tense then the body will regard the food as a poison. The physiology behind this is very sound, in that when responding to a stressful situation, all bodily processes will be diverted to cope with that, ie. the fight/flight response. At these times, the body is actually not designed to digest food. Digestion is also designed to begin in the mouth with the action of chewing so that juices are released to initiate the process, therefore by eating slowly and chewing our food adequately we allow the body to begin to make the most of the food. This simple action can be a contributing factor with many conditions of the digestive system. This reiterates the point about being **aware** and **conscious** of the food that we eat – it is impossible to **enjoy** food when anxious or in a hurry. This can lead to specific health problems, for example stomach ulcers and irritable bowel syndrome when the health of the body actually appears to be compromised by eating certain food in a certain way. The best advice would seem to be not to eat at all in these situations. For people with a busy work schedule, it can seem impossible to set aside a short time to be quiet and to eat but the benefits are usually well worth the effort.

Acid-alkaline balance

When food is metabolised, there is some residue which determines whether the environment of the body is acid or alkaline dominant. Depending on the chemical composition of this residue, the food is described as being 'acid-forming' or 'alkaline-forming'. This is not the same as the immediate chemical make-up of a food, for instance, an orange has a citric acid content but this is completely metabolised by the body with the resulting effect being to alkalise the body. The body is most efficient when it is alkaline-dominant and in order to achieve this, an ideal ratio of food intake would be 1/3 acid-forming food and 2/3 alkaline-forming food. As a general guide, most animal-products (concentrated proteins such as meat, fish cheese and eggs) tend to be acid-forming while most vegetables and fruit tend to be alkaline-forming (foods which can be eaten **raw** are particularly high in this list, especially the dark green vegetables, carrots and avocado pears).

This alkaline-dominance is the optimum state to be in, assisting the body to maintain good overall health. There are specific conditions which are related to over-acidity and the symptoms of which can often be eased by adopting a diet with a higher proportion of alkaline-forming foods (Holford, 1997). In fact, there is evidence to show that in the presence of certain health problems, real benefit can be achieved by 80% of the diet being alkaline-forming foods. These conditions include arthritis, irritable bowel syndrome, gastric ulcers, eczema, osteoporosis, tension headaches, anxiety states – any situation where there is an element of irritability or inflammation.

The benefits of raw food

The beneficial effects of a diet high in raw food are well documented over many generations and come from a variety of cultures with sources widespread throughout the world. For our species, as ancient hunter-gatherers, our diet would have been high in raw food (fruit, leaves and berries predominantly). In fact, 70% of the diet of a typical Westerner consists of foods that were unavailable during human evolution, namely dairy products, oils, refined sugars and salt. These foods are low in minerals and vitamins but high in fat and salt. There is evidence to show that these factors are linked to common western disorders including heart disease, high blood pressure, diabetes and arthritis. An American dentist, Weston A Price travelled extensively around the world from 1920 to 1940, studying the health of primitive societies. He discovered that, despite differences in the specific foods that they ate, the diet of people who were mainly free from mental and physical disease had one common factor: their food was simple, fresh and predominantly raw (Price, 1945).

When we eat raw food, we preserve its innate nutritional value allowing the body to access this for maximum benefit. In addition, we encourage and support the body to work as efficiently as possible. Cooked food is actually quite tiring to digest, as demonstrated when we feel really sleepy after a large meal. The Swiss physician, Max Bircher-Benner, was a great advocate of a raw food regime. He realised that important bodily processes, primarily those of the immune system, were employed to assist with the digestion of cooked food but not with raw food. He concluded that when we adopt a diet which is predominantly uncooked, then vital functions in the body can be released to protect and restore health (Kunz-Bircher, 1983). He realised that this vital energy can be released by simply starting every meal with some raw food. So, it may only need a few minor adjustments to introduce this vital element into everyday life, with the addition of fruit and/or salad at each meal.

The ability that raw food has to mobilise the immune system means that it is a valuable asset to use for conditions when this system is compromised, for example, when any infection is involved, when recovering from illness, for arthritis, and for more serious conditions such as cancer. In cases of fatigue, energy levels can be restored because minimal effort is required to digest the food and the body can utilise all it's resources effectively.

One major benefit of the addition of raw food is that the flavour of the food has not been diminished by the cooking process so that the taste buds get a real treat. If this way of eating is totally new, then it makes sense to introduce it gradually, slowly allowing it to become more and more a part of the daily routine. It is often surprising how easy this transition can be and people report a variety of positive responses including increased energy levels, improved skin condition, reduced incidence of headache and digestive problems, fewer infections and weight loss. What may at first seem quite a difficult regime turns out to be relatively easy with raw food becoming the ultimate in convenience food.

Anti-oxidants

We all have 'rogue cells' present in our bodies called free radicals, these cells, given certain conditions, can increase the risk of cancer and heart disease, inflammatory conditions such as arthritis and eczema as well as weakening the immune system. Latest information shows that 60% of cancer cells originate from free radical damage. The good news is that we can use substances called anti-oxidants to reduce the risk of these unruly cells taking over. Namely, anti-oxidants are Vitamins A, C and E and the minerals selenium and zinc. There are foods which minimise radical activity and discourage them from oxidising. Major sources are:

> Fish – mackerel and salmon
> Vegetables – avocado pear, cabbage, carrots, cauliflower, spinach,
> sweet potatoes and watercress
> Fruit – apricots, citrus fruits, grapes and mangoes
> All soya products.

Blood sugar levels

Certain foods cause blood sugar levels to rise dramatically giving a sudden burst of energy, unfortunately this is not sustained and it is followed by an equally dramatic drop, both in sugar levels and energy which then requires yet another boost to satisfy the increased demand. The body also seems to expect more and more each time, almost like a spoilt child. Stimulants which have this effect include chocolate, coffee, tea, cola and cigarettes.

Fluctuations in energy levels like this are tiring for the body, as its internal chemistry swings into action in attempts to restore balance, and can be avoided by introducing foods which initiate a more constant, stable environment. Foods which release energy in a steady fashion into the system are all fruits (releasing natural fruit sugars, especially bananas and dried fruit) and complex (ie. non-refined) carbohydrates, such as wholemeal bread, rice and pasta. Unstable blood sugar levels are often associated with feelings of tiredness, depression, headaches, feeling run down, continually catching minor infections and, for women, pre-menstrual syndrome and period pains.

Another factor which affects blood sugar levels is the amount of time between meals. If the time lapse is too long, energy reserves in the body begin to be drawn on and people can experience feeling shaky, dizzy or headaches. This would be the scenario if breakfast and then lunch are inadequate and hurried and then the evening is quite late. The situation is further compounded by trying to satisfy the inevitable hunger pangs, eating a quick snack of chocolate mid-morning and/or mid-afternoon. This is a vicious circle as blood sugar levels are further confused. To achieve a stable internal environment, the rule of eating '**little and often**' is the one to remember. A typical day would be:

- breakfast containing fresh fruit
- mid-morning snack (if needed) of fresh fruit
- lunch – making sure that this contains some fruit or salad
- mid-afternoon snack (if needed) of fresh or dried fruit
- **early** evening meal – again containing some salad or fruit.

Of course, as with all guidelines on diet and nutrition, the quantity of food eaten needs to be matched to the level of activity – in other words, only eat when you feel hungry. Busy, energetic people burn up the calories which need to be replaced. Exercise obviously affects sugar levels and this can often account for headaches experienced by some people after playing sport – particularly if their eating habits are irregular. This can be remedied by planning ahead and eating a sandwich or some fruit some time before (not too soon before).

Fluid intake

Two-thirds of the body consists of water, and it loses 1.5 litres of water per day via the skin, lungs, intestines and the kidneys, ensuring that toxic substances are eliminated. This obviously needs to be replaced from drink and food. Fresh fruit and vegetables consist of around 90% of water and they supply it in a form that is very easy for the body to use, as well as providing us with essential vitamins and minerals. Four pieces of fruit and four servings of vegetables can provide a litre of water, reducing the amount that needs to be taken through actual drinking; in fact an overload of liquid can place undue strain on the kidneys and increase pressure for both the circulatory and digestive systems. Reduce excessive fluid intake gradually. Try drinking from cups instead of mugs, you may be surprised to find that this is sufficient to satisfy your thirst, so why drink more? Recommended drinks are water, juices or herbal teas. The need for additional fluid intake will obviously be affected by consuming any processed food or food containing a high level of salt or seasoning in general.

Stress associated with food and nutrition

We all know that we can experience stress or tension in emotional, mental and physical ways. Each one of these aspects will then go on to affect, and be affected by, the others. Our bodies can feel internal stress caused by the way in which we eat. Also, the actual amount of food and drink that is consumed can contribute to this. If it is excessive then all the body systems will be under strain as it is processed. Basically, ingesting, digesting, assimilating and eliminating food is a demanding procedure and the more of it there is, the harder the body has to work. As a golden rule, the amount needs to be matched to activity and overall health, so a young, robust man who plays a lot of sport will obviously eat more and his body will happily cope with more than an older person who is mainly sedentary and whose health is not so strong.

Certain foods can also be more demanding on the body than others. Concentrated proteins, meat, eggs, cheese and milk are the most difficult to digest. While we need some protein for growth and repair, we need relatively small amounts in relation to other food types. The World Health Organization recommends 10% of total calories from protein, or about 35 grams of protein a day (Holford, 1998). Also, by reducing the intake of stimulants such as coffee, tea, sugar and chocolate we establish a kinder, gentler internal environment for ourselves.

We all know that stress comes from many sources in our lives and, it may be helpful at certain times, not to contribute further to this by the food that we eat. Also, the difficulty with stressful situations is the feeling of a loss of conscious control and, by making decisions about how and what we eat, we can maintain a sense of direction.

Nutrition to support the need for rest

To continue the theme of being kinder to ourselves via our diet, at times when the need for rest is indicated, we can support this with how and what we eat (refer to *Chapter 4*). This is appropriate during or after periods of illness or stress. Excessive food consumption can be overwhelming, and when someone is exhausted or upset, any food eaten will hardly be processed at all. To enable the body to recover and repair, it is essential to take in food which is not only easy to cope with so that vital energy can be used to restore health, but also contains the necessary nutrients to encourage this process. Recommended foods for this are, once again, the alkaline foods consisting of fresh fruit and vegetables. For maximum nutritional value these should be predominantly raw or just lightly cooked, with the addition of wholesome soups for ease of digestion. To avoid tiring and debilitating the body unnecessarily, intake of concentrated proteins should be kept to a minimum and ideally should consist of a small amount of fish. The ideal diet at this time being the traditional convalescent one so that the body can mobilise all its available power to assist recovery. Eating in this way can support whatever health care regime is chosen.

In addition to the **type** of food, the **quantity** needs to be considered and eating less is another way of resting, once again this enables the body to utilise all its available forces, no matter how limited, for the necessary job of recovery rather than for digestion. Small, well selected meals are the order of the day here.

For a healthy person restricting food intake, either partially or totally, as a fast has been proven to have benefits for the body's natural defence system. A 'user-friendly' way to introduce fasting into your life can be to have a modified fast for one day when you just eat fruit and drink juices or herb teas. This allows the system to feel cleansed and rested.

Anti-nutrients

The guidelines for these are simple, just avoid them. Prime anti-nutrients are salt and sugar. Salt is associated with high blood pressure, hardening of the arteries and contributes to the loss of valuable nutrients from the body. Salt attracts water and is a factor linked to cases of fluid retention. In addition, it disrupts calcium levels and is involved with degenerative conditions of the bones. The answer is to reduce any salt that you add to food gradually over a period of time and you will become used to the new taste. Just try it! Also, beware of added salt so read labels when you shop.

Refined sugar is also a 'non-food' in that it provides calories but absolutely no nutrition. Inappropriate sugar consumption is associated with heart disease, obesity, tooth decay, digestive disorders, headaches, depression and diabetes. It causes stress in the digestive system and the body has to work hard to sustain acceptable blood sugar stability. Humans are attracted to the taste of sweetness and it is difficult to break the habit of eating concentrated sweeteners. As with salt, the answer is to gradually reduce the sweetness in your food until you acquire new taste buds. In addition, you can substitute fruit which contains a natural simple sugar in the form of fructose, with bananas and dried fruit being the most efficient sources and, of course, they have high vitamin and mineral content.

Overweight

The market research company Mintel reports that one-sixth of women are trying to lose weight at any one time. Government reports show that 31% of men and 35% of women in the United States are defined as being clinically overweight, ie. they are 20% heavier than the average. The slimming industry in the West is enormous and there is a very familiar pattern of 'yo-yo' diets, as one impossible regime is broken after another. There are several important points to remember when planning any weight-loss diet:

- aim for a plan that is realistic so that it can be sustained
- match the eating pattern to your lifestyle so that you don't feel isolated socially
- always consider what you **can** eat rather than what you **can't**
- in order to lose weight you need to be taking in fewer calories than you use, so increase your activity level but make sure that the activity you choose is something that you **enjoy**
- increase daily exercise in a consistent, realistic way. For example, park your car slightly further away from the workplace, or use the stairs rather than the lift
- make sure that your diet is nutritious, high in fruit and vegetables and low in sugar and fat
- if you eliminate something that you are used to eating, remember to fill the void – in other words, plan a substitution, for example, take some fruit with you to work for the mid-morning snack so that it is easier to resist the doughnuts!
- use 'tactics' that work for you, maybe you eat from a smaller plate so that it still

looks like a big meal or you buy biscuits that you don't like so that you aren't tempted

- eat whole foods for their nutritional value and because your appetite will be satisfied with a smaller amount than if you eat refined foods
- eat **slowly** – primarily so that your body can digest the food efficiently, but also, so that you can eat smaller amounts without it being so obvious!
- remember that food and eating are to be enjoyed so avoid any feelings of resentment. Be human and allow yourself the occasional 'lapse'!

Self-help ways to improve digestion with massage, movement and breathing

Simple **self-help massage techniques** can assist with how the body deals with food, both for greater ease and efficiency. It can also relieve the most common form of abdominal pain, indigestion. Such a technique would be:

- lie down with a pillow under the knees. Take a few deep breaths
- place one hand on top of the other on the abdomen
- begin a smooth, continuous clockwise stroke using the flat of the hand. See *Figure 5.1.*
- 'scoop' from the lower to the upper abdomen, using the edge of each hand, one following the other. See *Figure 5.2.*

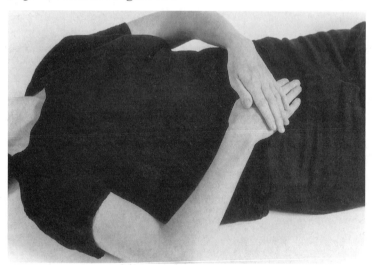

Figure 5.1

Breathing techniques are another way in which we can help the body to obtain the optimum amount of nourishment from our diet. In the same way that a fire needs air so too the body needs food and oxygen for energy. Adopting the basic three-part breath described in *Chapter 3 (p. 32)* is the most appropriate here.

Movement supports the body with it's natural processes for dealing with food. It can greatly relieve common problems such as indigestion, constipation, and heartburn. Gentle

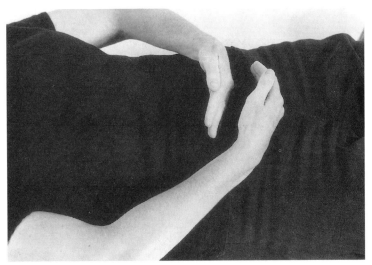

Figure 5.2

walking on a regular basis is often the most acceptable approach and the one that can be most easily fitted into the daily routine. Walking, along with massage and effective breathing assists the natural process of peristalsis, ie. the rhythmical contraction of the muscles of digestion to squeeze food gently through the system.

Yoga postures can be used to improve the function of all internal organs. There are specific postures which have beneficial effects on the organs of the digestive system, so that we can obtain with ease maximum nourishment from the food we eat . Two postures which gently massage the relevant internal structures are described in *Chapter 3*, the forward bend *Paschimottanasana* (*Figure 5.3*) and the spinal rotation *Ardha-Matsyendrasana* (*Figure 5.4*). See also *pages 23* and *27* .

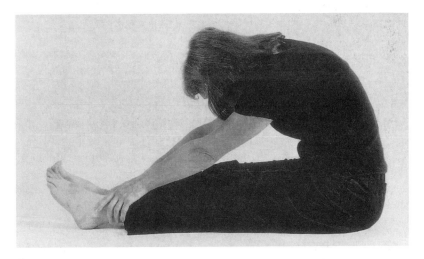

Figure 5.3

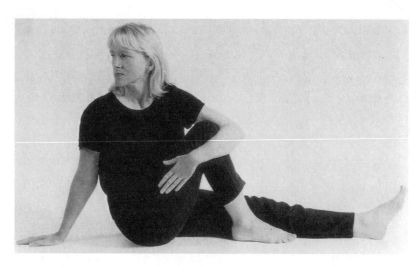

Figure 5.4

At-a-glance guide for nutritional advice with some common conditions

Arthritis – Reduce intake of acid-forming foods such as meat, cheese, milk and eggs. Increase intake of alkaline-forming foods including fruit and vegetables, especially dark green vegetables, carrots and avocado pears.

Fatigue – Maintain adequate blood sugar levels by eating fruit which releases natural sugar slowly. Eat regularly, avoiding long intervals between meals.

Fluid retention – Eliminate salt. Increase intake of fresh fruit and raw vegetables to discourage the accumulation of toxins.

Infections – Light meals, predominantly raw in response to the body's demand for rest.

Irritable bowel syndrome – Light, easily digestible food. Raw food at the beginning of each meal. Eat slowly. Practice deep breathing techniques.

Menopause – Increase intake of calcium rich foods such as sesame seeds, wholemeal bread and dark green vegetables. Reduce intake of concentrated proteins (meat, cheese and milk) as these create an acidic environment which then the body needs to re-balance by actually using up vital stores of alkaline substances, including calcium. Increase intake of phyto-estrogens (these are hormone-like compounds contained in certain foods) from soya, citrus fruits, wheat, liquorice, celery and fennel.

Migraine – Avoid long intervals between meals. Eat a light snack before exercise to prevent energy levels dropping. Avoid migraine 'trigger' foods – chocolate, cheese, red wine, citrus fruit and onions.

Pre-menstrual syndrome – Eat little and often to sustain blood sugar levels. Increase intake of foods containing Vitamin E – whole grains, dark green vegetables, nuts, seeds, avocado pears, sweet potatoes, watercress, tomatoes, vegetables oils, and mangoes and Vitamin

B6 – whole grains, beans, green leafy vegetables, cauliflower, nuts, bananas and fish.

Respiratory conditions – Avoid dairy foods because it encourages the formation of mucous.

Stress, anxiety and tension – Increase the proportion of acid: alkaline forming food to only 20% acid and 80% alkaline forming in order to reduce internal stress levels.

Summary

Hippocrates said,

> *Let food be thy medicine and medicine thy food.*

Our food is a very powerful medium and it can be used in a positive or a negative way to maintain and restore health. We can use our intuition with the food that we choose to eat and be guided by what the body needs. If you don't feel hungry, or if you can't smell the food (as happens when you have a cold), don't eat.

To summarise, the basic guidelines to apply to our diet and nutrition are:

- eat wholefoods
- aim for an acid:alkaline ratio of one third:two thirds
- eat at least five portions of fresh fruit and vegetables daily
- match eating habits to **your** lifestyle
- eat **consciously**, being aware of what and how you are eating
- see food as a source of vital energy – aim to eat some raw food daily
- eat **slowly** – try to be the last person to finish the meal!
- remember that eating is primarily a **sociable** activity – choose the company!
- drink only when thirsty
- eat only when hungry
- reduce salt and sugar intake
- have a rest occasionally with a mono-fast, ie. the same type of food for one day
- **enjoy** eating, enjoy occasional treats, avoid any guilt feelings. Remember you are only literally 'spoiling' yourself when these cease to be occasional
- be kind to yourself
- have fun with food – at every stage, from the shopping and selection, to the preparation, right through to the eating.

References

Blythman J (1996) *The Food We Eat*. Michael Joseph Ltd, London: 277

Holford P (1997) *The Optimum Nutrition Bible*. Piatkus, London: 97

Holford P (1998) *The Optimum Nutrition Bible*. Piatkus, London: 36

Kenton S, Kenton L (1995) *The New Raw Energy*. Vermilion, London: 29

Kunz-Bircher R (1983) *The Bircher-Benner Health Guide*. Unwin, London: 75

Price Weston A (1945) *Nutrition and Physical Degeneration*. Price-Pottenger, Nutrition Foundation Inc

6

Massage

Massage is something that we all do naturally. We instinctively rub an aching shoulder or a child's knee when they fall over or we reach out to touch a friend who is troubled. The medium of massage is touch and there is increasing evidence to show the therapeutic value of touch. The sense of touch is the most heightened sense when we are born, as new-born babies rely on the tactile sensations of holding, suckling and caressing. Touch is so central to our well-being that without it we can become depressed, anxious and irritable. The dictionary definition of **touching** is, 'the action of feeling something with the hand etc', the operative word here is **feeling**, touch involves not only a sensation but also an **emotion**.

Massage can be used to reinforce our need for touch in a non-threatening, reassuring, supportive way within comfortable limits. Therapeutic massage assists the normal functioning of the body and reduces anxiety states. Everything in nature is designed to move, our movement is essential to health and can, in itself, be described as a form of massage. Massage treatments co-operate with this innate desire for activity and the strokes themselves follow the movements of the body. It has been used throughout history by many cultures. Ancient Chinese, Indian and Egyptian manuscripts refer to the use of massage for prevention and treatment of illness. In Europe there are many references within Roman and Greek societies. In the present day, research studies in Sweden with Kindergarten children have shown that regular massage reduces levels of hyper-activity and encourages sociability.

Given the establishment of trust and co-operation, massage is appropriate for all ages and it can be used to relieve physical and emotional discomfort. It is a form of communication, being all the more powerful because it is **beyond words**, engaging with us on an intuitive level. This enables the body to respond truly without the need for sophistication .

Professional treatment

There are times when the need for a professional treatment is indicated; you may feel that you need the knowledge, care and advice of a practitioner. Massage is now firmly established as an effective therapy; a consultation providing it with a safe, supportive environment. The treatments can be applied to a variety of situations, either to restore or to maintain overall health, to reduce tension which is held in the muscles in response to a physical or emotional threat or to assist with recovery from injury. The effects on the body include:

- soothing the nervous system
- manipulation of muscles
- circulation of the blood and lymphatic fluid assisted
- improved lung function
- enhanced skin condition
- a beneficial influence on digestive and cardiovascular functions
- promotion of relaxation
- increased sense of well-being, many people report an increase in energy levels.

Massage at home

Massage has both technical and human elements, each to varying degrees and it can be experienced either in a professional setting or in a home environment. There is a strong tradition of natural therapy which comes from a culture of home care. There are many massage opportunities to support fitness and to promote relaxation which can be applied to family and friends. Home care and self-help techniques can extend the beneficial effects of a professional treatment.

Hand massage

We use our hands constantly and they inevitably feel tired and stiff at times. Giving a hand massage is so convenient and there is none of the nervousness that can accompany a full body treatment. Obviously it has benefits for the hands themselves, but also, it reduces overall nervous tension and promotes deep relaxation.

1. **Soothing strokes**. Hold hand, palm up, in one hand. Stroke palm of hand with your other hand, down to wrist and back again (*Figure 6.1*).
2. Turn hand over. Stroke over back of hand with your thumbs (*Figure 6.2*).
3. **Thumb pressures**. Using your thumbs, press all over the back of the hand.
4. Repeat soothing strokes (*Figure 6.3*).
5. **Finger massage**. Hold the hand palm down and work each finger in turn. Gently stretch each one from the base to the tip. Use circular pressure around each joint and then rotate the finger first in one direction and then in the other (*Figure 6.4*).
6. Open out the palm. With the palm facing up, stretch the palm using a fanning stroke with your thumbs. Hands are often held closed in and this movement reverses that position, releases tension and feels very welcome and comforting (*Figure 6.5*).
7. Repeat original soothing strokes.

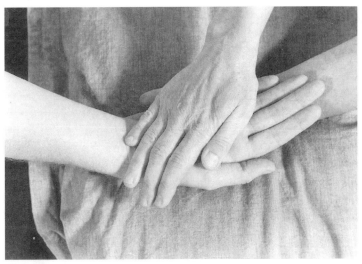

Figure 6.1

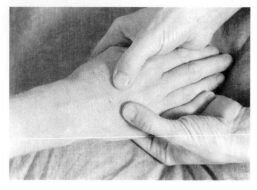

Figure 6.2

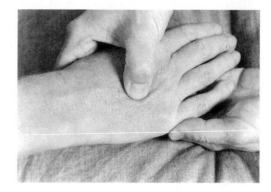

Figure 6.3

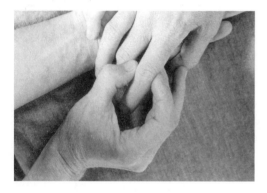

Figure 6.4

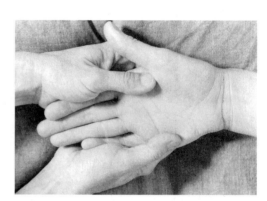

Figure 6.5

Each of these strokes can be repeated several times, you may wish to concentrate on some more than others – be guided by your intuition and by the ones that are received with the most delight.

Foot massage

The bones, ligaments and muscles of the feet are not more robust than those of the hands yet they are continually expected to carry heavier loads than any other part of the body. In addition, they are often subjected to cramped conditions. We are all familiar with how discomfort of our feet affects the entire body, the sentiment expressed in the relentless cry of 'my feet are killing me'. Foot massage relaxes and revitalises not just the feet but also the entire body.

All of the foot treatments mentioned here divert the body's attention to the feet and away from the head. They can be used to relieve congestive symptoms such as headaches, eye strain and anxiety. They also all play a valuable role in restoring energy and recuperation after a period of illness.

The ideal position to receive foot massage is to be lying down, or sitting in a comfortable chair, with the legs and feet completely supported. To give the treatment, work first one foot and then the other. Use a firm touch so as to avoid any ticklish response.

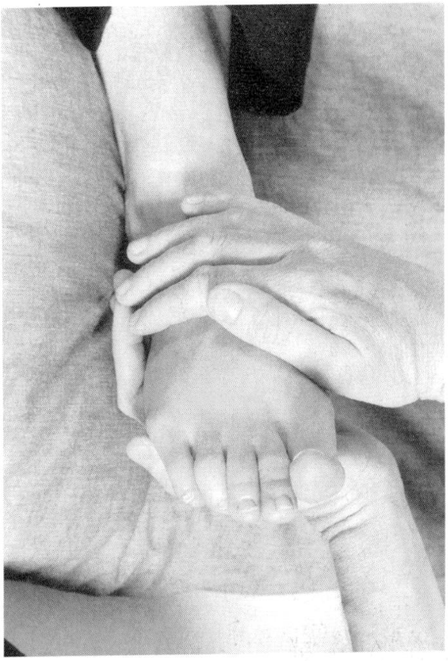

1. Hold the foot between your hands and stroke the foot firmly from the toes to the ankles. Return the hands to the toes with a light stroke (*Figure 6.6*).
2. Support the foot with both hands, fingers underneath and thumbs on top. Use a fanning stroke from the base of the toes up towards the ankle. Slide back to the toes (*Figure 6.7*).
3. Toe massage. Use a circular pressure around each toe and rotate it in both directions. Gently pull each toe (*Figure 6.8*).
4. Knuckling. Make a fist of your hand and place the knuckles on the sole of the foot at the base of the toes. Use a firm pressure down towards the heel (*Figure 6.9*).
5. Fingertips. Use a very light fingertip pressure moving randomly over the whole of the sole of the foot (*Figure 6.10*).
6. Movement. Hold the heel in one hand and, with the other hand, flex the foot up and down. Rotate the foot, first in one direction, and then in the other (*Figures 6.11a,b*).
7. Finish with the original soothing stroke.

As with the hand massage, each of these strokes can be repeated at your discretion.

Figure 6.6

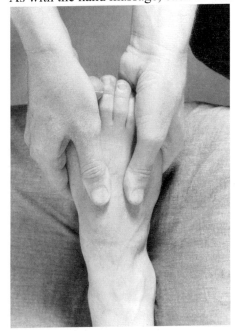

Figure 6.7

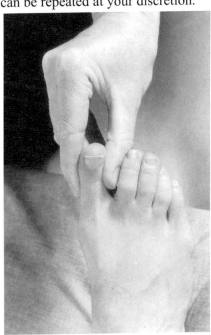

Figure 6.8

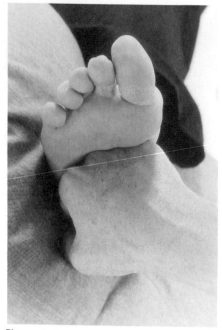

Figure 6.9

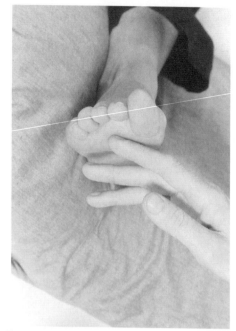

Figure 6.10

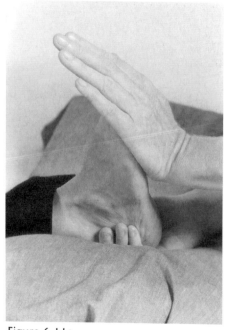

Figure 6.11a

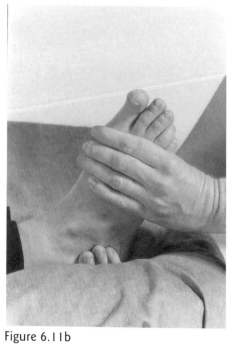

Figure 6.11b

Self-massage of the feet

Rocking and rolling

Standing for long periods of time is tiring for the entire system, tension is held in the muscles, circulation is restricted and pressure is felt in the lower half of the body. An easy exercise to alleviate this is rocking back-and-forth from heel to toe (*Figures 6.12 a, b*).

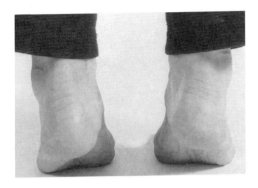

Figure 6.12a

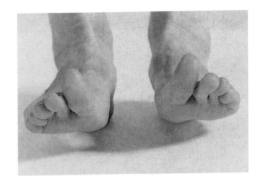

Figure 6.12b

Sitting down, place a ball under each foot and roll the foot backward and forward (*Figure 6.13*).

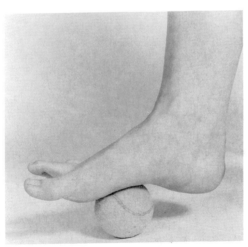

Figure 6.13

Water therapy

Dewy grass – The pioneer of hydrotherapy, the use of water for the purpose of encouraging natural healing, was Father Kneipp, a Bavarian priest. He recommended walking barefoot through dewy grass as being beneficial for many illnesses and for maintaining health.

Paddling – This simple, yet effective treatment is stimulating and energising, it increases body tone, improves circulation and develops resistance to infections. Fill the bath with ankle-deep cold water.

Paddle in the water for two minutes. Dry the feet with a warm towel.

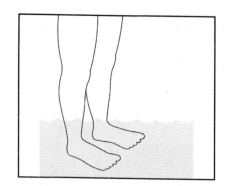

Showers – This is an excellent tonic for the nervous system, it increases circulation and, by diverting blood from another part of the body, it relieves congestion elsewhere. In the shower, direct cold water to the soles of the feet for one minute.

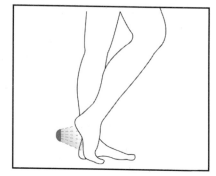

Additional home care applications for hydrotherapy

For insomnia – When sleeping is difficult because of an overactive mind, this procedure can be very beneficial. Quite simply, it diverts the body's attention away from the head.

- turn on the cold water tap and place each wrist under the running water for one minute
- lightly mop the wrists dry with a warm towel. Go back to bed, breathing deeply and being aware of the increased warmth in your hands.

For anxiety, stress or panic – This simple exercise works with the body's natural processes by taking attention away from the part of the nervous system whose job it is to respond to action and, instead, connects to the nerves that promote a relaxed, calm state. It can be used at home, at work – anywhere in fact where there is a supply of cold water.

- splash cold water all around the eyes for one minute. Lightly pat dry with a warm towel.

Abdominal massage

This self-massage can be for the relief of any abdominal discomfort, to ease the digestive process and for overall relaxation. Self-treatment is often most welcome as most people feel unsure about being touched here. For detailed descriptions of the procedure refer to *Chapter 5, p. 52.*

Neck and shoulder massage

Neck and shoulder massage given in the sitting position can reduce muscular tension, subdue headaches and alleviate feelings of stress and anxiety. It is a most popular site for tension and people speak about 'having the weight of the world on their shoulders'. This short massage sequence is perfectly adaptable, it can easily be fitted into a busy lifestyle and, because it can be administered through clothes, it can take place either in the home or the work environment. The person to be massaged sits in a chair, with you standing behind.

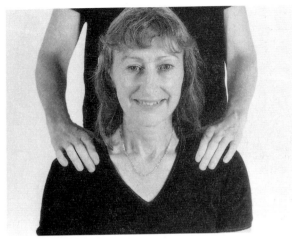

Figure 6.14

1. Stroking – light strokes from the sides of the head down the neck and over the shoulders (*Figure 6.14*).
2. Kneading use open hands to alternately squeeze and release the muscles. Work on both shoulders and the tops of the arms (*Figure 6.15*).
3. Circular strokes – stroke in a circle over the shoulder, one hand following the other (*Figure 6.16*).

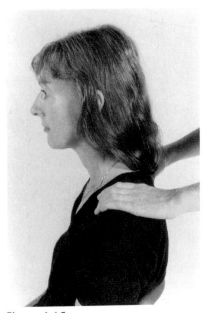

Figure 6.15

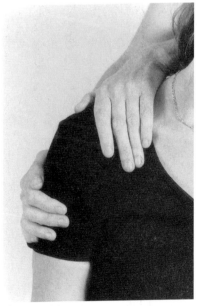

Figure 6.16

4. Thumb pressures – work on the ridge of the shoulders, using firm thumb pressure from the centre to the outside (*Figure 6.17*).
5. Repeat light soothing strokes.
6. Hacking – with relaxed hands hack across the shoulders and upper back. Allow the hands to bounce up and down from relaxed wrists (*Figure 6.18*).
7. Repeat light soothing strokes.
8. Neck – stand at the side and hold the forehead in the palm of one hand. Lightly squeeze up and down the neck using circular thumb pressures, with fingers and thumb either side of the spine (*Figure 6.19*).
9. Repeat soothing over the head, neck and shoulders.

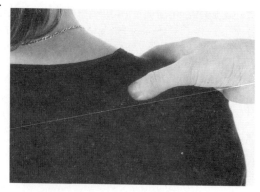

Figure 6.17

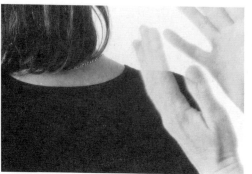

Figure 6.18

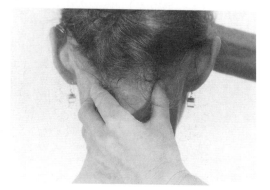

Figure 6.19

Baby massage

It is a natural response to stroke and caress babies, providing mutual pleasure and delight for both parent and child. A daily massage allows time for the unique relationship to develop away from the day-to-day routine of caring for the baby. In addition, there is increasing evidence to show that massage is beneficial for the baby's physical and emotional health. It can be used to relieve specific conditions such as colic, constipation, irritability and restlessness. It has the added bonus of reducing the parent's anxiety at times when they may otherwise have been feeling helpless.

The therapeutic benefits of baby massage have been extensively documented and there is increasing evidence to support this. Tiffany Field of The Touch Research Institute in Miami is at the forefront of this research. In 1984 she conducted a study in a group of premature babies who were massaged over a period of ten days. The results showed that these babies had a 47% greater weight gain than babies who were not massaged. At a follow-up study one year later, these same babies achieved higher development scores.

In the home environment no special techniques and no definite sequence is necessary. You will probably find that the soothing strokes are the most appropriate but be guided by what your hands want to do naturally and what the baby enjoys – he/she will undoubtedly let you know! If you wish to use any medium at all, then a light vegetable oil (almond or sunflower) is best. But it is not essential and, for babies with extra sensitive skins it is better to use nothing at all. It is further enhanced by being an enjoyable experience, being lead entirely by the baby, when he/she is ready, with lots of eye contact and using games and rhymes.

1. ***Legs*** – Begin the massage with the legs as an easy introduction, away from more
    sensitive parts of the body.
    Hold the baby's foot in one hand and stroke from the thigh to the toes with the other
    hand (*Figure 6.20*).

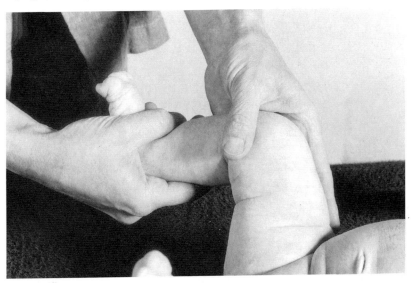

Figure 6.20

Gently massage the leg using a wringing movement down the full length of the leg towards the toes (*Figure 6.21*).

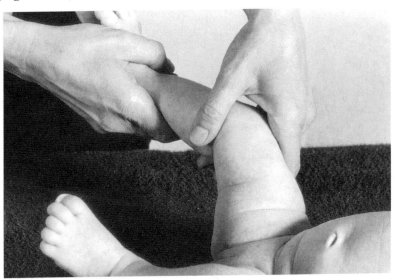

Figure 6.21

Squeeze and rotate each toe, stroke the whole of the foot (*Figure 6.22*). Repeat with the other leg.

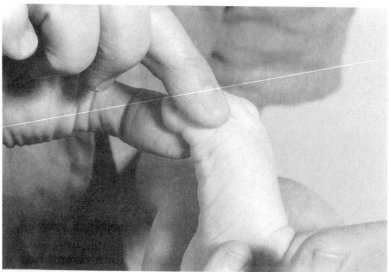

Figure 6.22

2. **Arms** – Hold the baby's hand and stroke from the shoulder to the fingers with the other hand (*Figure 6.23a, b*).

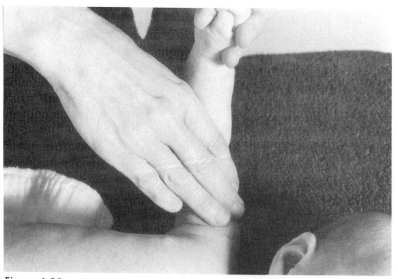

Figure 6.23a

Gently massage the arm using a wringing movement down towards the hand (*Figure 6.23b*).

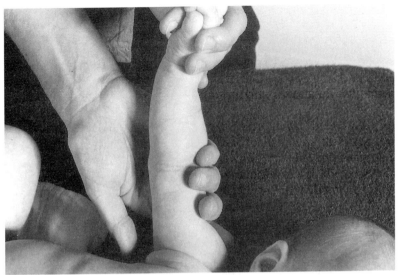

Figure 6.23b

Stroke the baby's hand and, as it begins to relax, squeeze, rotate and gently stretch each finger in turn (*Figure 6.24*).

Repeat with the other arm.

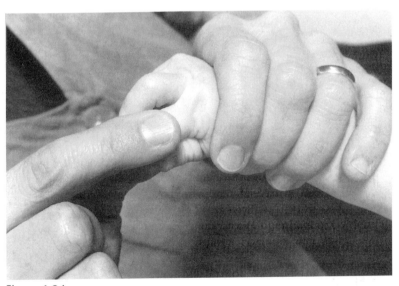

Figure 6.24

3. ***Abdomen*** – now that the baby is relaxed and settling into the session, you can proceed to more sensitive areas. Using the flat of your hand, stroke from one hip diagonally across the body up to the opposite shoulder. Repeat to the other side (*Figure 6.25*).

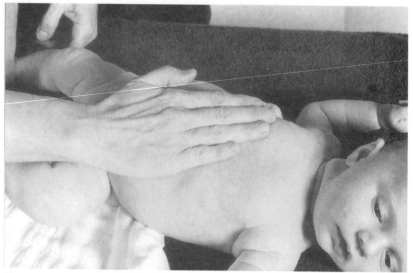

Figure 6.25

Stroke clockwise over the abdomen, one hand following the other. This can relieve colic and stomach ache (*Figure 6.26*).

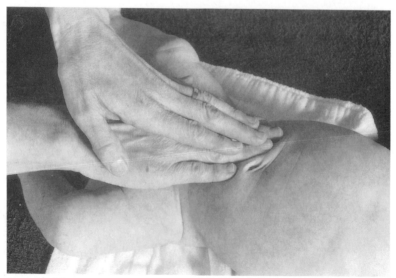

Figure 6.26

4. ***Chest*** – Place both hands over the navel, stroke up the centre of the chest, spread your hands out and over each shoulder and smooth down the arms to the hands (*Figure 6.27*).

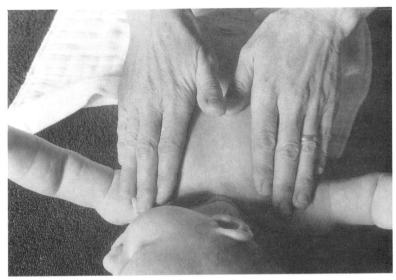

Figure 6.27

5. ***Back*** – Turn the baby to lie onto his/her front. Please note that for very small babies, this can be with the baby lying across your lap. With one hand following the other, stroke down the full length of the body from the base of the neck to the toes.
    Using gentle circular pressure, place the thumbs either side of the spine and work up towards the neck (*Figure 6.28a*).

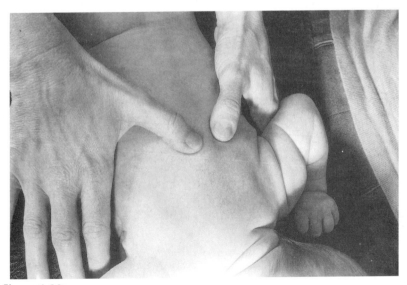

Figure 6.28a

Finish by gliding first one hand down the length of the body and then the other, gently alternating from one to the other (*Figure 6.28b*).

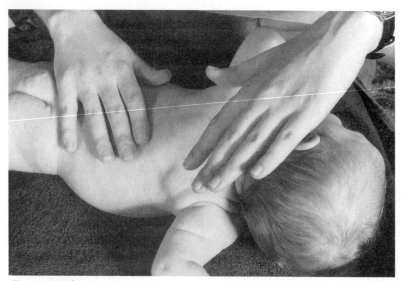

Figure 6.28b

Passive movements

Babies enjoy this opportunity to move and stretch away from the restrictions of clothes.

1. *'Cycling'* – Holding the babies feet, gently bend each knee towards the body, alternating from one leg to the other. This can often relieve colic and constipation as the movement encourages intestinal activity (*Figure 6.29*).

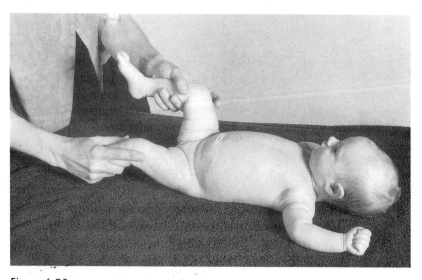

Figure 6.29

2. ***Arms*** – Take hold of the baby's hands and place them on the chest, then gently stretch them wide out to the side (*Figure 6.30*).

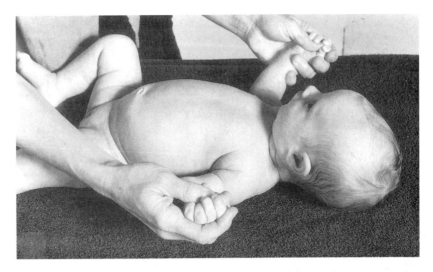

Figure 6.30

3. ***Alternate arm and leg*** – Hold the opposite hand and foot. Bring them to touch each other and then open them out again, stretching them as much as the baby allows. Repeat to the other side (*Figure 6.31*).

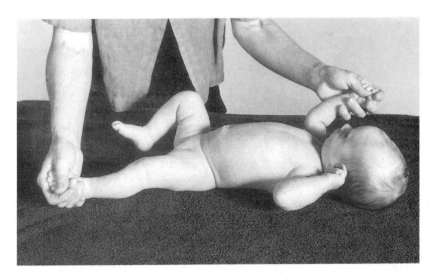

Figure 6.31

Summary

Health care need not always be a struggle, ideally it also involves the ability to relax and feel good about yourself. Massage facilitates this approach. At the same time, an optimum state of health and well-being is not necessarily personified by being calm all the time. The important element here is to be able to feel, to be aware of our feelings and, at times, to be able to express these feelings spontaneously. Massage is one way to achieve this greater awareness.

7

Pregnancy and post-natal care

The wonder of pregnancy is that, despite the millions of babies born each day, each one is unique and each set of prospective parents will have their own expectations and priorities. Many women aim to be as fit, strong and prepared as possible, so that they are completely involved in their choice of health care at this crucial time. Health care supports this approach, providing ways to meet the inevitable demands while still reinforcing the fact that pregnancy is a natural event. This chapter looks at some of the ways in which this can be achieved. Expectant parents can plan the progress and manner of the pregnancy, the birth itself and the postnatal care in ways to suit them.

One way to define stress is to say that it is a response to change and pregnancy is certainly a time of great changes. There are obvious **physical changes**, not least of which is the need for great reserves of stamina and endurance skills, but there are equally huge **emotional** changes too. Even when the pregnancy is planned and wanted it is a stressful time as the changes have to be not only adapted to, but also welcomed and embraced. Contributing to the stress levels is the mixture of excitement and apprehension surrounding the imminent birth, the apprehension about the unknown being greater for first-time parents.

Pregnancy is, thankfully, never an isolated event. During those vital nine months, normal and natural life circumstances take place. Pregnancy is part of the scenario of inevitable life situations; some pleasant, some not so pleasant, some stressful, some predictable and some totally unexpected. These events may involve relationships, families, careers, finances, travel – in fact everything that adds to the rich pattern of life. The pregnancy may affect, or be affected by, some of these situations. Parallel to this situation, the woman is adapting to the demands of the pregnancy, which can be all encompassing and often is all that she **wants** to focus on.

Yoga for mothers and babies

The practice of yoga encompasses the holistic approach using physical movements (asanas), breathing and relaxation techniques in order to establish a sense of awareness and integration within each individual. This resonates particularly with pregnancy, birth and the time immediately after birth, which are all times of change, adjustment and growth on all levels of being. Many of the classical yoga postures and relaxation procedures seem to be tailor-made for the experience of pregnancy and many others can be adapted to suit individual need.

Support

Yoga supports the desire that many pregnant women have to feel more in control physically, emotionally and spiritually . It brings a sense of connection within the self and also with the baby, so that they can both feel prepared and in an optimum state of health at such a vital time. One important principle in the practice of yoga is that attention and stability (Sanskrit: *Sthira*) and ease and pleasure (*Sukha*) can exist in the body side by side (Feuerstein, 1990). This is helpful during pregnancy, post-natally and during the birth itself. To carry, deliver and care for a baby, a woman needs to be strong in every way. It is equally obvious that relaxation would be beneficial at these times too. Yoga teaches that a sense of power and of being at ease are both equally important and, that they are especially advantageous when acting together. Stability means power and control, not stress, and ease means relaxation and rest, not weakness.

Yoga during pregnancy can be practised by women who already have it as part of their lives, or by women who are coming to it for the first time. The common bond between pregnant women provides great support in a class situation. This creates an ideal environment in which to practice yoga with a partner. Pairs yoga, where the mother and a partner work together with postures, can be especially beneficial and enjoyable during pregnancy, providing direct physical and emotional support. When the partner is the baby's father this can introduce another dimension to each of the relationships – between the couple and between the individuals. They are physically together, aware of each others' movements and, in a gentle, easy manner, they are already a family.

In the vital post-natal period exercise and movement need to be introduced gently and appropriately, gradually becoming more adventurous as each woman feels ready. Yoga easily lends itself to this since it is a naturally progressive practice. It provides a shared activity between the mother and the baby which can be a welcome break from the day-to-day routine care. Moving and stretching at this time can be pleasurable – and moderately challenging too – as the woman begins to 'reclaim' her body again. The baby can join in as he/she grows and begins to demonstrate remarkable flexibility. The baby's father can also become involved with pairs yoga; providing a positive involvement in the early days with a new baby.

Practice during pregnancy

The mountain posture (*Tadasana*) is particularly relevant during pregnancy. This involves standing with awareness so that the weight of the body is evenly distributed. The ankles, knees and hips are in alignment, the arms hang loosely at the side, shoulders are wide and relaxed and the chin is level (*Figure 7.1*). This employs the principle previously described of stability and relaxation existing synergistically within the body; standing tall with awareness of the strength and control of the large structures that are essential to support both the mother and the baby and, also, by creating a feeling of space and breathing deeply, benefiting from feeling relaxed and at ease. Specifically, *Tadasana* can help to alleviate lower back pain which often occurs during pregnancy by extending the spine tall and free through the centre of the body. This posture adds to the comfort of both mother and baby. The simplicity of *Tadasana* means that it can be practised almost anywhere.

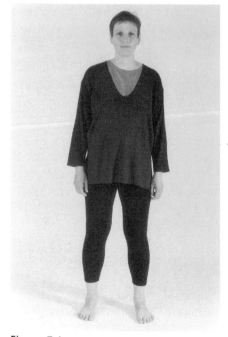

Figure 7.1

The cobbler pose (*Baddha Konasana*) improves circulation to the pelvic floor, encourages the natural widening of the pelvis and tones pelvic floor muscles. These muscles carry the additional weight of the pregnancy and all women are so aware of this pressure, often from the earliest days. The woman sits with soles of her feet together, knees wide and relaxed, holding on to her toes. See *Figure 7.2*. Please note that care must be taken with this posture if there is hyper-flexibility of the ligaments around the sacro-iliac joint. For continued practice of this posture, perhaps it can be adopted as an alternative position when relaxing at home?

Simply by the action of **squatting**, the pelvic structures are gently encouraged to widen so it is obviously fitting to include this in a yoga pregnancy programme. Gravity comes to the baby's assistance here helping her to assume the optimum position

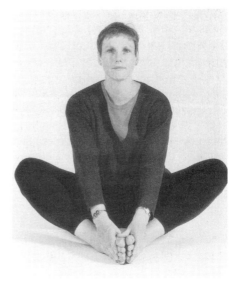

Figure 7.2

during life in the womb and, in labour, it eases entry into the world. It does, however, require strong leg muscles to hold this posture for any length of time so it is advisable to devote time to this posture during pregnancy. With feet slightly wider than the hips, the woman squats down encouraging the knees to stay in line with the toes. Once again, there is an awareness of space with the spine extending tall and the shoulders feel wide open and relaxed. This posture encourages the natural elasticity of the pelvic floor muscles. This position is often instinctive during labour, feeling open and releasing (*Figure 7.3*). The action of squatting can be further enhanced by the assistance of a partner (*Figure 7.4*), so that the entire length of the spine can feel both free and stretched. This posture reduces strain on the structures of the lower back and brings relief to back pain which many pregnant women experience.

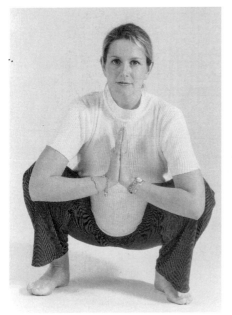

Figure 7.3

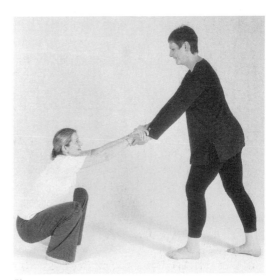

Figure 7.4

A gentle version of the cat posture (*Marjaraiasana*) is invaluable at this time. This involves kneeling on all fours, breathing in while gently looking up (*Figure 7.5a*) and then, on an out-breath, gently rounding the spine (*Figure 7.5b*). The 'hammock' of muscles of the abdomen which cradle the baby are strengthened and toned. Again it helps to make both mother and baby feel comfortable. The whole of the pelvic region is gently massaged. Also, it can reduce lower back tension and the baby is encouraged, by gravity, into the favourable anterior position. In the hollow spine position, *Figure 7.5a*, care should be taken not to over-extend the abdominal muscles. If time is limited, the cat posture is probably the most valuable single posture and great benefit can be obtained by practising it on a daily basis, just for a few moments.

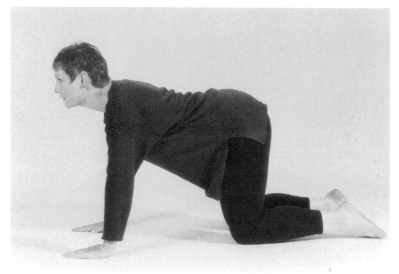

Figure 7.5a

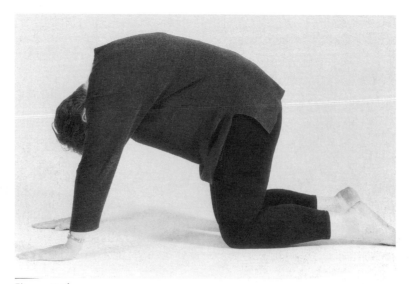

Figure 7.5b

The warrior posture (*Virabhadrasana*) strengthens the thigh and back muscles which are so important when carrying, and also deliverying, the baby. The woman stands with feet apart turned to one side, inhales and extends the arms wide to shoulder height (*Figure 7.6a*), exhales and turns to one side (*Figure 7.6b*), inhales and extends the arms over her head, exhales and bends the front knee (*Figure 7.6c*). Again, there is a feeling of space as the spine extends tall. The nature of this posture is such that it promotes feelings of being assertive, confident and strong – all useful emotions to experience in preparation for labour. Breathing techniques can be easily and naturally applied within asanas; these are often instinctively called on later during the actual birth. When breathing in, there is a sense of energy and strength and, when breathing out, there is a feeling of relaxation and ease.

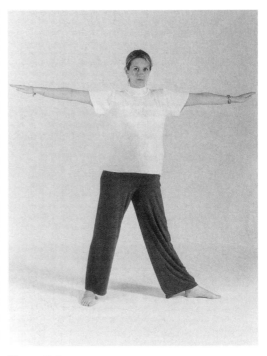

Figure 7.6a

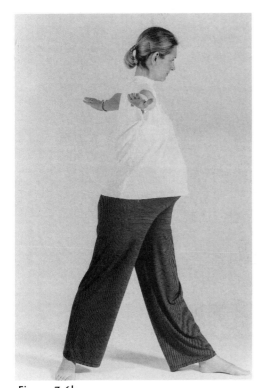

Figure 7.6b

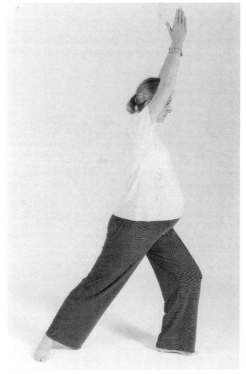

Figure 7.6c

Taking into account the increased weight during pregnancy, which averages 11.9kg by the 40th week, it is desirable to relieve the potential pressure whenever possible. Classical inverted yoga postures can be adapted to achieve this, by using the floor and wall for support. The woman lies on the floor on her back with legs against the wall. There is no weight-bearing of the body so she can be totally relaxed and feel completely supported. In this way gravity is used to drain away any excess fluid which may have accumulated in the legs. Depending on the position in which the baby is lying, a support may be occasionally needed under the lower back for additional comfort (*Figure 7.7*). Within the home environment, the time spent in this posture can be enjoyably extended by listening to favourite music and using it as a time to relax.

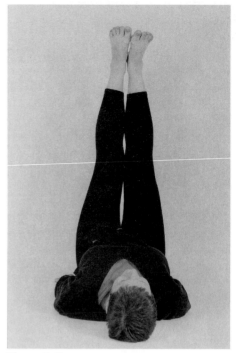

Figure 7.7

As the pregnancy becomes more advanced, the muscles of the lower back can become strained and painful. Partners can help to alleviate this with a simple seated posture (*Figure 7.8*). The supporting partner's feet are placed close against the woman's lower back so that she can lean back against them. If the baby's father is the partner, giving this support is a very exclusive time being an experience that not only the couple can share, but also, that the three of them share together. In this practical way the couple can share any burden and strain of pregnancy. The actual practice of yoga, by its very nature, can be enriching, needing no words of explanation.

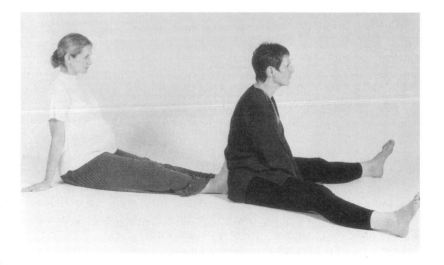

Figure 7.8

Relaxation plays an important part within standard yoga practice and this is especially so during pregnancy. However, the classical position of lying prone needs to be adapted for comfort. The woman lies on her side using cushions to support herself and the baby (*Figure 7.9*). This quiet time provides the mother with an opportunity to focus on the unique existence of the baby and on the special relationship already established between herself and her child. It reinforces the yoga session as a shared activity, either being able to be completely quiet and still if that is how the baby chooses to be, or alternatively, a time to rejoice in energy and life if he/she decides to be active. Standard yoga breathing techniques support relaxation and, as previously mentioned, are often valuable friends during the actual birth, reinforcing an atmosphere of positive control. Each inhalation restores energy and vitality. The exhalation is particularly important establishing a sense of release, a 'letting-go' of tension and discomfort; this provides an opportunity for rest and recovery.

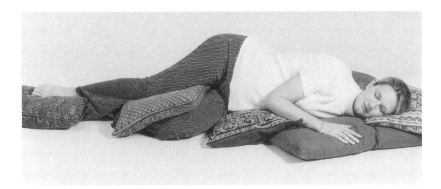

Figure 7.9

Post-natal care

Yoga can be significantly beneficial post-natally when a woman is coming to terms with her new identity, both on a physical and an emotional level. It is enjoyable to be able to move and stretch without the additional weight of the pregnancy. If the woman has practised yoga during her pregnancy, to be able to continue with familiar postures having her baby now beside her is very reassuring. Gentle practice supports the process of recovery, repair and adjustment. Sharing the yoga with her baby makes a statement about the life that they have together and also the life that they have as individuals. Many of the familiar postures from pregnancy still apply and there are some which can be aimed specifically at this time.

The **cat posture**, previously described, is helpful for toning up all the muscles and structures which have been working so hard during the previous months. When it is appropriate to increase the movements, usually after approximately six weeks, a further stretch can be added. This involves extending each leg in turn on the inhalation and then bringing it through towards the head on the exhalation. See *Figures 7.10a* and *b*. This can be particularly helpful if practised on a daily basis and, although time is at a premium with a new baby, by setting aside just a few minutes each day, there will be long term rewards.

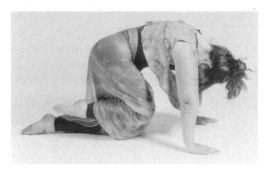

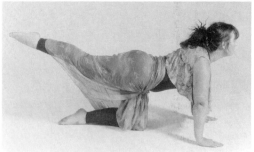

Figure 7.10a   Figure 7.10b

To assist with the repair of the pelvic floor muscles, continued practice of the **cobbler pose** is encouraged. This posture can be shared with the baby as he/she begins to grow and demonstrate his/her flexibility. See *Figure 7.11*.

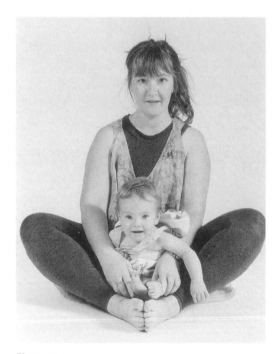

Figure 7.11

Caution at this time is necessary when practising certain postures. While many of the suggestions described here can be safely followed throughout pregnancy, post-natally the guidance of a teacher is recommended. In particular, **forward bending poses** tend to compress healing structures in an unhelpful way. An ideal way to achieve this movement, without compression, is by flexing each leg in turn towards the chest, while reclining. See *Figure 7.12*.

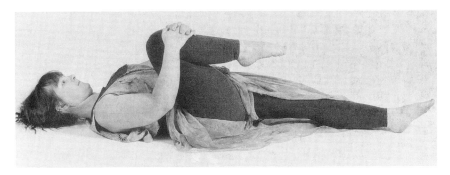

Figure 7.12

Yoga practice is an ideal way to enjoy moving and stretching together away from the daily routine. As the baby grows, he/she can discover a new range of movement. Both the baby-yoga and the partner-yoga can provide a way for father-involvement at this vital time when relationships are developing.

Relaxation for the new mother is obviously essential and beneficial for the entire family. Opportunities for this may be rare and need to be taken whenever possible. New babies can often share in this by appreciating the close contact. See *Figure 7.13*.

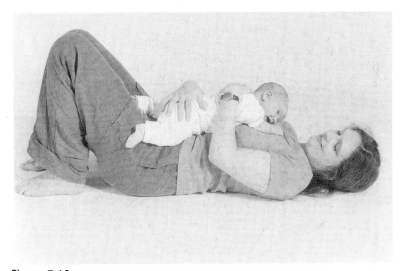

Figure 7.13

Yoga is an enjoyable way for a woman to actively manage her pregnancy. Also, in conjunction with help from health care professionals, yoga offers a supportive and restorative influence in post-natal care. In fact, yoga supports the entire experience of pregnancy, birth and parenthood. Classical principles relate perfectly to the entire process. There is an opportunity for the whole family to feel, at each stage, supported and strengthened and, equally, restored and rested.

Massage during pregnancy

A gentle massage during pregnancy can be very constructive and enjoyable. Not only by promoting relaxation, but also, it can relieve some of the common symptoms of pregnancy such as, back ache, cramp, neck and shoulder tension and insomnia. All the strokes should be smooth and gentle, with no deep pressure massage. If the person giving the massage is also the baby's father this allows him to feel more involved in the pregnancy and it is another way in which the new family spend time together.

It is important that the woman feels comfortable during the massage so, depending on how advanced the pregnancy is, she may have to adapt her position. She may be lying down with pillows to support her back, or lying on her side with pillows to support the abdomen, or perhaps sitting astride a chair leaning on a cushion (*Figure 7.14*)

Areas of the body which respond particularly well to massage at this time are the back, neck, shoulders and legs. Understandably, women are often anxious about having the

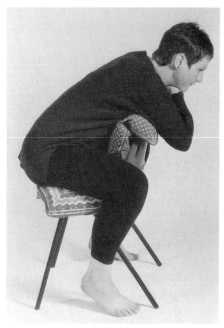

Figure 7.14

abdomen itself massaged, however, a very gentle circular stroke here can reduce feelings of pressure and tightness. A self-massage is often a good option so that the woman can choose how much pressure to apply.

Back massage

Backache is probably the most common and, most troublesome complaint during pregnancy. A massage can relieve much of the unease, also note that taking a warm bath and deep breathing exercises are often beneficial.

1. ***Stroking***. Place your hands on the lower back with thumbs either side of the spine. Smooth the length of the spine with relaxed hands, out across the shoulders, glide down the sides of the body and repeat. See *Figure 7.15*. The touch needs to be gentle but definite and, in fact, be guided by your partner as to how much pressure to use.
2. ***Alternate hands***. This is still stroking, but using the hands alternately. One hand strokes upwards as the other strokes downwards. See *Figure 7.16*.
3. ***Diagonal stretch***. This helps to relieve pain in the lower back caused by the necessary pelvic adjustments needed to facilitate the birth. Start with both hands in the centre of the spine, stroke firmly away towards one shoulder with one hand and to the opposite hip with the other hand. Repeat to the other side. See *Figure 7.17*.
Repeat the initial soothing stroke.

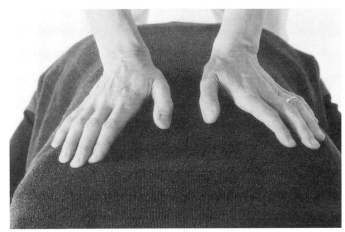

Figure 7.15

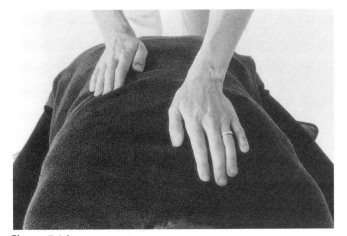

Figure 7.16

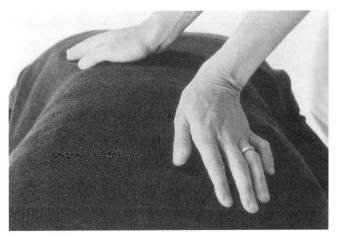

Figure 7.17

Leg massage

This can relieve swelling and pain in the legs and reduce pain and discomfort caused by varicose veins and cramp. The additional weight and pressure caused by the pregnancy inevitably means that the legs become tired and stressed.

1. ***Soothing strokes*** – With the woman lying down with her back and legs supported, smooth up either side of the leg, over the knee (crossing over the hands) and down again to the ankle (*Figure 7.18*).

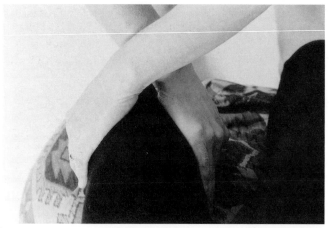

Figure 7.18

2. Back of leg – using the flat of your fingers, push firmly up from the back of the heel towards the back of the knee, one hand following the other. Repeat immediately so that it feels like a continuous movement. See *Figure 7.19*.
3. Repeat initial smoothing strokes.

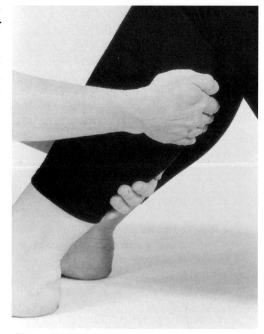

Figure 7.19

Neck and shoulder massage

This is the sequence described in *Chapter 6, pp. 63–64.*

Massage during the birth

During the birth itself, the **back** massage can be particularly helpful. Psychologically it is calming and reassuring, and physically, it relieves backache. In addition, the **foot massage** described in *Chapter 6 (p. 58)* can greatly relieve the pain of the contractions.

It is important to note that each birth is unique and, it is vital to be guided by what the woman actually wants. Often, in complete contrast to what had been planned beforehand, the woman cannot bear to be touched in this way. This reaction is not to be taken personally.

Post-natal massage

Massage after the birth can help to alleviate some of the stresses and strains of new parenthood. Physically the body has received a major trauma and it needs time to repair. Massage can also assist with the 'roller coaster' of emotions felt at this time, as the mother can feel alternately blissfully happy and then full of anxiety about the implications of parenthood. Not least, the massage gives the mother some much-needed care and attention.

Nutrition during pregnancy

The most crucial time for optimum nutrition is actually before conception, this ensures the most favourable conditions for the future baby's growth and development. If nutrition needs to be upgraded at this time, general guidelines apply, see *Chapter 5* .

For pregnant women, as with everyone, appetite needs to be matched to activity. It is not necessary to increase the **amount** of food consumed but to 'listen' to the body and simply to eat when hungry and when the idea of food is appealing.

There are specific problems associated with pregnancy which sometimes can be alleviated from a nutritional angle:

Morning sickness

- eat concentrated protein foods (meat, eggs, cheese, milk) in moderation
- some people find relief in the Chinese remedy for nausea, ie. ginger. Tea made from fresh grated ginger root can be helpful
- be guided by your intuition and eat what you feel that you can
- eat little and often.

If all else fails, you can comfort yourself with the thought that new research suggests that morning sickness is a natural mechanism designed to protect unborn babies from food poisoning at a time when a woman's immune system is compromised. This does not explain why some get it more than others and why so many women suffer given modern food hygiene standards, but it may be of some comfort.

Constipation

Contributing factors to this are, (a) because the increased weight falls forward in the body there is a loss of abdominal tone and, (b) the additional weight in the pelvic cavity presses on the colon causing impaired function. This problem can be alleviated by ensuring adequate intake of fresh fruit and vegetables, making these raw if possible. In addition, you can reduce the pressure on the colon by practising the squatting exercise described earlier (*p.75*).

Heartburn

There are many old wives tales attached to heartburn and they are worth a try because one of them may work for you. You may wish to try food combining, ie. eating little and often and, not eating protein foods with carbohydrates (bread, pasta, rice, potatoes). This kinder way of eating is sometimes what the digestive system needs (Doris and Jean, 1984).

Eating in the advanced stages of pregnancy

Again be guided by your intuition and eat as, and when, you feel the need. Most women report only being able to eat very small, simple meals at this stage. This may be because they feel that, due to the increased pressure in the abdominal cavity, they have very little room to spare or because they are responding to the impending birth in an instinctive manner. Animals prepare in the same way, they sense the imminent injury and they know that they will heal better if their body is free to handle the trauma rather than having to use vital energy to digest food. Be reassured, knowing that adequate food stores have been laid down during the previous months.

Hydrotherapy

Hydrotherapy is defined as 'the use of water to encourage natural healing'. All life begins in water, so we can resonate easily with it as a natural healing environment. It lends itself easily to home-use and it is reliable, safe and pleasant. Various methods are used in the application of water, these include immersion, splashing and moist compresses. There are some basic statements to support its rationale:

- cold water limits blood loss from small blood vessels
- cold water reduces pain of pressure and inflammation
- cold water is reassuring
- cold water keeps an injury supple. Moisture stops the tissues from drying out and prevents irritation
- cold water encourages elimination by relaxing the skin
- hot and cold water provide a gentle massage effect
- hot water can re-direct blood flow from congested areas. By applying heat to the non-injured area attracts blood and reduces pressure at the injured site
- water is economical and ecological.

Hydrotherapy during pregnancy

Paddling

As described in *Chapter 6* (*p. 62*) this self-massage of the feet is extremely beneficial for promoting efficient circulation. In pregnancy it can be used to reduce pressure in the lower part of the body and to relieve pain caused by varicose veins.

Method – run a bath with ankle-deep cold water. Walk up and down the bath. Start with 30 seconds on the first day and gradually increase this to two minutes.

Hydrotherapy during labour

* Spraying the face – Use an atomiser to spray cold water, directing to the forehead. Obviously this is immediately cooling but also, by stimulating the nervous system, it aids concentration and reduces anxiety.

* Cold neck compress – wring a towel out in cold water, roll it up and place around the neck. This relieves tiredness and encourages deep breathing.

* Hot compress on lower back – place a hot towel against the lower back. This relaxes the pelvis between contractions.

* The birth pool – some women elect to use a birth pool, the advantages being that during labour floating eases pressure on the spine and the pelvis is freer. Floating in the warm water promotes relaxation and relieves the intensity of the pain.

Hydrotherapy immediately after the birth

If the birth is treated simply as a physical injury, there can be no doubt that it is a major trauma for the body and the application of water can be especially relevant.

* Cold compress to the perineum – Immediately after delivery of the placenta, place a towel wrung out in cold water under the pelvis, bring up between the legs and lay across the abdomen. Replace as the towel dries for the next 48 hours. This treats the injury to the tissues of the perineum (the 'floor' of the pelvis), bleeding is arrested but elimination is not stopped and the overall shock to the body is reduced. The woman is also encouraged to rest at this time.

Conclusion

It is so important for prospective parents to be able to plan and to make informed choices about the management of the pregnancy and about the nature of the birth and post-natal care. These choices reflect their individuality and ensure their unique involvement. However, a small word of caution is necessary here. Exactly because each birth – and each baby – are totally unique, no-one can predetermine its progress. It is sometimes necessary to change plans at the last minute due to unforeseen circumstances. The new plans being in the best interests of all concerned. It is helpful to build in, as part of the plans, the need to be flexible and adaptable. If the best-laid plans have to go awry, what does that matter when you have all the magic and wonder of a new baby?

References

Feuerstein G (1990) *Encyclopedic Dictionary of Yoga.* Paragon House, Location: 350–352

Grant D, Joice J (1984) *Food Combining for Health.* Thorsons, New York

Mitchell S (1998) *Naturopathy – Understanding the Healing Power of Nature.* Element Books, Shaftesbury: 81

Review – how to use this book

The suggestions contained in this book can be used whenever appropriate, according to need, practicality, and personal preference. Each one can be used in isolation or combined together in a variety of permutations. There follows a list of common conditions to illustrate this. These are just examples; as your confidence grows, you will be able to trust your intuition and apply the skills to each new situation. Your attention will, quite rightly, be on the symptom but, ideally, this is to be seen as the starting point so that you can then consider wider, more positive, long-term, preventative issues. These may raise questions such as:

How does this make me feel and does that remind me of anything else in my life?

For example, if there is an irritation, perhaps there is another aspect of your life that is irritating you?

Why has this happened just now?

It is often significant with migraine attacks, for example, that they are probably the only way to make busy, highly motivated people actually **stop**.

How can I prevent this situation happening again?

The process of attaching a **meaning** to the problem, of self-reflection, brings with it greater understanding and awareness so that it is possible to begin to address the reason behind the situation. In this way, we can move forward in a positive manner. It may be that other symptoms arise but these can, in turn, be viewed in the same way. We are all dynamic individuals, responding to life situations. Each step can be seen as a process of growth so that, strange though it may seem, we can make the most of our health problems and learn from them.

We may, by answering these and similar questions, realise what is contributing to the problem but, realistically, not always be able to change the situation. Sometimes the realisation in itself is enough to help, as though the understanding was all that was needed.

Natural health care programmes for some common conditions

Anxiety:
* Use hydrotherapy treatment around the eyes (*p. 62*).

Arthritis:
* Adopt a low protein diet, avoiding acid-forming foods. Increase intake of alkaline-forming foods (fresh fruit and vegetables).
* Massage and/or reflexology for stress control and pain relief.
* Introduce appropriate exercise on a daily basis. This may be a gentle walk or sitting and practising hand and foot exercises.
* Deep breathing exercises to assist with the elimination of toxins.

Asthma:
* Avoid dairy food because of its ability to produce mucous.
* Deep breathing exercises to improve lung function.
* Massage and/or reflexology to reduce stress. Asthma causes, and may be caused by stress, so to reduce this is helpful in the long-term.

* Yoga exercises to improve lung function, especially the Triangle and Cobra postures (*pp. 22, 25*)

Back pain:
* Regular yoga practice, under supervision initially. This will strengthen the muscles that support the spine so as to prevent problems in the future.
* Self-help reflexology for pain relief.
* Massage for gentle mobilisation.

Breathing difficulties:
* If these are associated with anxiety, use the hydrotherapy treatment of cold water splashes around the eyes (*p. 62*).

Constipation:
* Deep breathing exercise to provide an internal massage, being aware of a relaxed expansion on the inhalation and a retraction of the abdominal muscles on the exhalation.
* Yoga exercises, especially those to improve intestinal tone – the spinal rotation, the forward bending posture and the cat pose – as described in *Chapter 3*.
* Gentle inversion to remove any tension or compression in the abdominal cavity (*pp. 29–32*).
* Increase intake of fresh fruit and raw vegetables.
* Only drink when thirsty. Excessive fluid intake will weaken intestinal tone.
* Self-massage of the abdomen (*p. 52*).
* Self-help reflexology especially of the reflex for the large intestine (*p. 14*).
* Squatting exercises. As a self-massage technique for the appropriate muscles (*p. 75*).
* Eat slowly to assist efficiency of the digestive process. Aim to be the last person at the dinner table to finish eating! Avoid eating if angry/hurried/tense.
* Instinctively, we often transfer our emotions to the digestive system so, emotionally, consider what else in your life makes you feel tense or congested?

Cramp:
* Deep breathing exercises to promote adequate oxygenation so as to eliminate acidic toxins. Visualise fresh, healthy blood healing and nourishing the effected area as you breathe.
* Reduce intake of acid-forming foods (concentrated proteins) and increase intake of alkaline-forming foods.

Fatigue:
* Increase intake of fruit and vegetables to boost consistent energy levels.
* Reduce intake of foods which take vital energy from the body to be digested (concentrated protein and processed foods).
* Eat 'little and often'. Avoid eating late at night.
* Introduce regular exercise to boost energy levels.
* Take a rest . Enjoy and appreciate it.
* Reflexology or massage treatments.

Fluid retention:
* Eliminate salt totally from the diet. (Salt attracts water.) Increase intake of raw food to encourage the body to eliminate excess fluid.
* Inversion of the body so as to use gravity to reverse the effects of sluggish circulatory and lymphatic systems (*pp. 29–32*). In addition, whenever possible, rest with the feet raised.

* Self-help reflexology to stimulate drainage of excess fluid (*p. 15*).
* Regular yoga practice for exercise and to improve all body functions.
* Massage treatments.

High blood pressure:

* Avoid excess fluid intake, this will put extra strain on the kidneys and increase pressure within the body.
* Yoga practice, initially under supervision, to promote relaxation.
* Massage – for rest and relaxation.
* Reduce intake of stimulants, such as tea, coffee and alcohol.
* Eat foods which your body can easily digest (fruit, vegetables, soup, fish) so as to avoid causing any undue pressure.
* Take some time to walk each day.
* Deep breathing exercises to reduce feelings of stress and tension.

Infections:

* This is the body asking for **rest**. Preserve your energy to fight the infection.
* Eat raw food, fruit and vegetables, so that you can 'free up' the immune system to concentrate on fighting the infection.
* If, as in the case of a cold, you can't smell, then don't eat. This is your body saying that it is not attracted to food. Again this will allow the immune system to work at it's most efficient. The next day introduce a small intake of raw food.
* Self-help reflexology. Focus on the relevant area, for instance, in the case of a sore throat, work the throat reflex (*p. 11*).

Insomnia

* Use hydrotherapy treatment of cold water application to the wrists, (*p. 62*).

Irritable bowel syndrome:

* Eat **slowly** to encourage adequate digestion.
  Deep breathing exercises – for massage of the internal organs.
  Eat raw food at the beginning of every meal to ensure efficient digestion
* Self-reflexology. Especially for the large intestine (*p. 14*).
* There is usually an element of stress with IBS, so regular yoga practice would address this. In addition, certain postures would reduce tension and compression in the abdomen, this would be any inverted postures. Some postures improve abdominal tone, these include forward bending ones and spinal rotations (*p. 23; pp. 27–28*).
* Massage to provide relaxation.
* You could ask yourself if you feel irritated and, if so, what causes that irritation?
* Avoid large meals especially late at night.

Menopause:

* Increase intake of foods rich in phytoestrogens and calcium rich foods (*p. 54*).
* Massage and/or reflexology treatments for relaxation and support.
* Yoga for relaxation.
* Self-reflexology to aim to restore balance within the system and to relieve symptoms such as hot flushes and anxiety.
* Deep breathing exercises to relieve some of the symptoms, such as insomnia and tension.

Menstrual problems:

* Gentle inversion of the body to reduce feelings of congestion in the pelvic cavity (*p. 31*).This can be practised daily in the week prior to menstruation.

* Yoga to encourage a state of balance within the body. The Cat pose described on *page 28* is especially helpful for painful/irregular periods.
* Self-help reflexology to assist with pain relief.

Migraine:

* Maintain even blood sugar levels – increase intake of natural sugars in fruit and reduce intake of stimulants such as chocolate, coffee and tea. Avoid long intervals between meals. Try to avoid 'dips' in blood sugar after exercise by eating a light meal one hour before the activity.
* Self-massage of the feet and hydrotherapy techniques to relieve pressure from the head (*pp. 58–62*).
* Avoid possible 'trigger' foods, eg. cheese, chocolate, red wine and oranges. Self-reflexology to relieve headache (*p. 9*).
* Massage for relaxation.
* Yoga as a way of managing stress.
* The headache may be the external presentation of toxins in the system. Deep breathing exercises will help to eliminate these toxins.
* Try to see the migraine as a 'friend'. It makes you rest and take time out of a busy schedule. Perhaps you find it difficult to rest without a reason? If this sounds familiar, perhaps you could think about alternative ways to rest and relax.
* Often people who frequently have migraine headaches are perfectionists who are always striving for the impossible. Does this should familiar?

Neck tension

* Massage – professional and/or home care.
* Yoga to reduce overall tension.
* Self-help reflexology on the neck reflex (*p. 10*).

Overweight

* Increase exercise levels within realistic limits and choose an activity that you enjoy.
* Reduce intake of fats and sugar.
* Increase intake of fruit and vegetables. Reflexology treatments – to stimulate the metabolism.

Poor circulation

* Self-massage of the feet with hydrotherapy (paddling in cold water). See *page 62*.
* Deep breathing. Visualise warmth and energy being taken to the hands and feet with each inhalation.
* Increase intake of raw food so that no vital energy has been lost by the cooking process.

Pre-menstrual tension:

* Maintain steady blood sugar levels (increase intake of fruit and eat small meals, avoiding long intervals between meals). Substitute fruit for snacks instead of cakes and biscuits.
* Eat adequately in the middle of the day.
* Eat foods rich in Vitamins E and B6 (*p. 54*).
* Self-reflexology to reduce stress.
* Massage treatments to promote relaxation and to provide an exclusive rest time.

Pregnancy:

* See *Chapter 7, p. 73*.
* See advice under specific conditions, for instance, varicose veins and high blood pressure.

Sinusitis:
* Avoid dairy products to reduce congestion.
* Regular reflexology sessions supported by self-treatments on the sinus reflexes (*p. 12*).
* Yoga breathing exercises.

Varicose veins:
* (This condition often occurs during pregnancy when the increased weight, and resulting pressure, inhibits the efficiency of venous activity.)
* Deep breathing exercises to facilitate effective circulation
* Leg massage (*p. 84*).
* Home care – Hydrotherapy (paddling in cold water to encourage improved circulatory function) (*p. 62*). In addition to this, spray the lower leg with cool water from the ankle up to the knee.
* Inversion exercise to relieve pressure on the lower limbs (*p. 30*).

The important principle here is to use an approach that feels comfortable and appropriate for you, and one that fits in with your lifestyle. You may choose to make certain changes and discover new aspects of yourself on the way but that is the challenge.

Summary

What this book has attempted to show is how everyone can, if they wish, use natural health care, to some degree or other. Most people's first introduction is when they arrange to see a practitioner in a professional environment. It is a familiar scenario for someone to come for consultation almost as a last resort, saying, 'I have tried everything else, so now I am trying this'. It is as though the symptom has brought them to the therapy. This apparently negative situation often becomes a very positive one during a course of treatments as the recipient grows to feel more involved with their health care. The practitioner acts as the reference point and they (the client) feels better resourced as a result of the treatment. Their understanding and awareness about how they are feeling increases. Instead of just wanting to get rid of a problem, they begin to enjoy looking after themselves, this is made easier by the fact that often the treatment itself is a pleasant experience. This attention and care promotes increased confidence so that self-help applications in the home environment take on a higher profile. This way we work with the wishes and intelligence of the body, rather than against them. As a system, the body strives to be well; that is the state it prefers to be in which we can help it to achieve. Natural health care provides ways to feel better. This practical everyday use of natural health care extends the quality of the treatment sessions and increases self-esteem still further. The increased understanding and resulting clarity is sometimes enough, in itself, to ease the problem and to have a beneficial effect on overall health status.

The choice of therapy does matter in that the individual concerned needs to relate to it, to enjoy it and to feel comfortable with it. In the professional setting, they also need to relate to the practitioner so that a relationship of mutual trust and respect can be established. From then on, the consultation becomes the forum enabling a process of health care to take place, almost regardless of the medium of the therapy itself.

Holistic health care illustrates that sickness is not an unfortunate accident but a way of communicating within the body and with the world around. To attach meaning to how we are feeling physically, emotionally and spiritually presents a challenge which may not always be easy – and perhaps it won't always happen. In response to this reflective process, it may be necessary to make changes in factors that are influencing our health. However, each of us can initiate these changes as, and when, we feel ready.

This approach enables us to make the most of being unwell; this doesn't mean that we need to enjoy the illness, but rather, that we accept it as part of ourselves and try to see why it has happened and how to move forward and, hopefully, prevent the same set of circumstances happening again. This way relieves the pressure of striving to be well all the time. Our health reflects our life and, as such, it is never going to present with a consistently perfect scenario. Health doesn't have to be in extremes of either being ill or being completely well but instead we can be responding to how we feel at any one time.

Rather than simply responding to illness, the complementary health care approach offers ways to gain insight into how we function as full, rounded, complex individuals. This is a continual process, reflecting our human nature and the 'ups and downs' that form part of the glorious, varied, rich pattern of life.

If you allow a natural health care regime to become part of your life, you can choose what format this takes. Give yourself time to look after yourself and always remember that you are worth it. Feel inspired, use your imagination and use ways that feel appropriate for you. Let your judgement be the guide as to the manner of the care; at different times you may feel that it needs to be comforting, relaxing, supportive, healing, stimulating, gently provoking or innovative. Trust yourself because,

...you know best.

Recommended reading list and useful addresses

Bircher R (1961) *Eating Your Way to Health*. Faber, London

Blythman J (1996) *The Food We Eat*. Michael Joseph, London

Buchman DD (1994) *The Complete Book of Water Therapy*. Keats Publishing, New Canaan, Connecticut, USA

Ernst E (ed) (1996) *Complementary medicine – an objective appraisal*. Butterworth-Heinemann, Oxford

Holford P (1998) *100% Health*. Piatkus Books, London

Holford P (1997) *The Optimum Nutrition Bible*. Piatkus Books, London

Jack A (1999) *Let Food be Thy Medicine*. One Peaceful World Press, Becket, Massachusetts

Kent H (1995) *The Complete Yoga Course*. Headline, London

Kenton L, Kenton S (1994) *The New Raw Energy*. Vermilion, London

Kunz-Bircher R (1981) *The Bircher-Benner Health Guide*. Unwin Paperbacks, London

LeShan L (1974) *How to Meditate*. Harper Collins, London

Maxwell-Hudson C (1988) The Complete Book of Massage. Guild Publishing, London

Mitchell S (1997) *The Complete Illustrated Guide to Massage*. Element Books, Shaftesbury

Mitchell S (1998) *Naturopathy – Understanding the Healing Power of Nature*. Element Books, Shaftesbury

Montague A (1986) *Touching - The Human Significance of the Skin*. Harper and Row, London

O'Brien P (1991) *A Gentler Strength*. Thorsons, London

Shapiro D (1990) The Bodymind Workbook. Element Books, Shaftesbury

Swami Satyananda Saraswati (1969) *Asana, Pranayama, Mudra, Bandha*. Bihar School of Yoga, 1969

Thomson CL (1968) *A Commentary on Foot Fitness*.T.K. Publications, Edinburgh

Williamson J (1999) *A Guide to Precision Reflexology*. Quay Books, Mark Allen Publishing Ltd, Salisbury

Useful addresses

School of Complementary Health
38 South Street
Exeter EX1 1ED
Tel: 0044 (0)1392 499360
Fax: 0044(0)1392 410954
email: jan.sch@breathemail.net
website:
www.schoolofcomplementaryhealth.co.uk

Association of Reflexologists
27 Old Gloucester Street
London WC1N 3XX
Tel: 0870 567 3320

Axelsons Gymnastiska Institut
Gastinkegatan 10–12
Box 6475
113 82 Stockholm

British Wheel of Yoga
25 Germyn Street
Sleaford
Lincolnshire NG34 7RU
Tel: 01529 303233
email: office@bwy.org.uk
website: www.bwy.org.uk

Federation of Precision Reflexologists
38 South Street
Exeter EX1 1ED
Tel: 01392 499 360
email: jan.sch@breathemail.net

Touch Research Institute
The University of Miami Medical School
Miami
Florida

Index

A

abdominal massage 62
acid-alkaline balance 47
anti-nutrients 51
anti-oxidants 48
anxiety 25, 62, 89
Ardha-Matsyendrasana 27
arthritis 48, 54, 89
asanas 21
  ~ cat (Marjaraiasana) 28, 76, 79
  ~ cobbler (Baddha Konasana) 75
  ~ cobra (Bhujangasana) 25
  ~ half-spinal twist (Ardha-Matsyendrasana) 27
  ~ mountain (Tadasana) 74
  ~ forward bend (Paschimottanasana) 23
  ~ Shoulderstand (Sarvangasana) 29
  ~ triangle (Trikonasana) 22
  ~ warrior (Virabhadrasana) 77
asthma 89

B

baby massage 64
back ache 82
back massage 82
back pain 29, 36, 90
Baddha Konasana 75
Bayly 5
Bhujangasana 25
birth 81, 85
breathing 32, 52
breathing difficulties 90
Buddhists 5

C

cancer 48
career 3
cat posture 28, 76, 79
cheese 50
chocolate 48
cigarettes 48
circulation 29, 92
climate 3
cobbler pose 75
cobra 25
coffee 48
cola 48
conception 85
constipation 14, 86, 90
consultations 3
contractions 85
cramp 82, 90
culture 2–3

D

deep breathing 22
de-tox 34
digestive disorders 36
digestive problems 3, 29
disposition 3

E

eczema 3
eggs 50
energy
  ~ of the body 6
environment 3
exercise 3

F

fatigue 54, 90
first aid 8
fluid intake 49
fluid retention 15, 54, 90
food 44
foot care 18
foot massage 58
forward bend 23
free radical damage 48

G

genetically modified foods 46
gravity 29

H

half-spinal twist 27
hand massage 57
headache 3, 9, 36
heart conditions 36
heartburn 86
heredity 3
high blood pressure 4, 36, 91
Hindus 5
holistic health care 95
home care 8
hormonal imbalances 36
hormones 21
hydrotherapy 86
  ~ for feet 19

I

immune system 48
infections 4, 54, 91
insomnia 62, 82, 91
internal organs 23
inverted yoga postures 78
irritable bowel syndrome 54, 91

L

leg massage 84
lifestyle 2–3
lungs 25

M

Marjaraiasana 28
massage 52, 56–57, 59–61, 63, 65, 67, 69, 71
  ~ abdominal 64
  ~ during birth 85
  ~ during pregnancy 82
  ~ hand 57
  ~ leg 84
  ~ neck and shoulder 63, 85
meat 50
media 44
meditation 36, 39
menopause 54, 91

menstrual disorders 28–29
menstrual problems 91
migraine 54, 92
milk 50
morning sickness 85
movement 52
muscles 23
Muslims 5

N

natural health care 95
neck and shoulder massage 63, 85
neck and shoulder tension 82
neck pain 10
neck tension 92
nutrition 3, 44
~ during pregnancy 85

O

organophosphates 46
overweight 51, 92

P

paddling 62
pain relief 13
pairs yoga 74
panic 62
parenthood 81
partners 78
Paschimottanasana 23
passive movements 70
post-natal care 73, 75, 77, 79, 81, 83, 85,87
posture 34
precision reflexology 8
pregnancy 28, 73, 75, 77, 79, 81, 83, 85, 87, 92

pre-menstrual syndrome 54
pre-menstrual tension 92
proteins 50

R

raw food 47
reflexology 5, 9, 11, 13, 15, 17, 19
~ precision reflexology 8
relationships 3
relaxation 19, 36–37, 39, 41, 43, 79
relaxation techniques 37
respiratory conditions 55
respiratory disorders 36
rest xii, 4, 36–37, 39, 41, 43
rotation postures 26

S

salt 51
Sarvangasana 29
selenium 48
self-help advice xi
self-massage
~ of the feet 61
shoulder tension 17
shoulderstand xii, 29
showers 62
sinusitis 12, 93
skin conditions 36
sore throats 11
Sphinx 26
spinal tension 22
spine 25–26
squatting 75
stamina 73
Sthira 74
stress 25, 50, 55, 62, 73

sugar 51
Sukha 74
support 73

T

Tadasana 74
tea 48
tension 10
three-part breath 32
Touch Research Institute 64
triangle pose 22
Trikonasana 22

V

varicose veins 93
Virabhadrasana 77
visualisation 36, 38
vitamins 48

W

water therapy 61
whole food 46

Y

yoga 21, 23, 25, 27, 29, 31, 33, 35
~ for mothers and babies 73
~ inverted postures 78

Z

zinc 48